Affirmative Mental Health Care for Transgender and Gender Diverse Youth

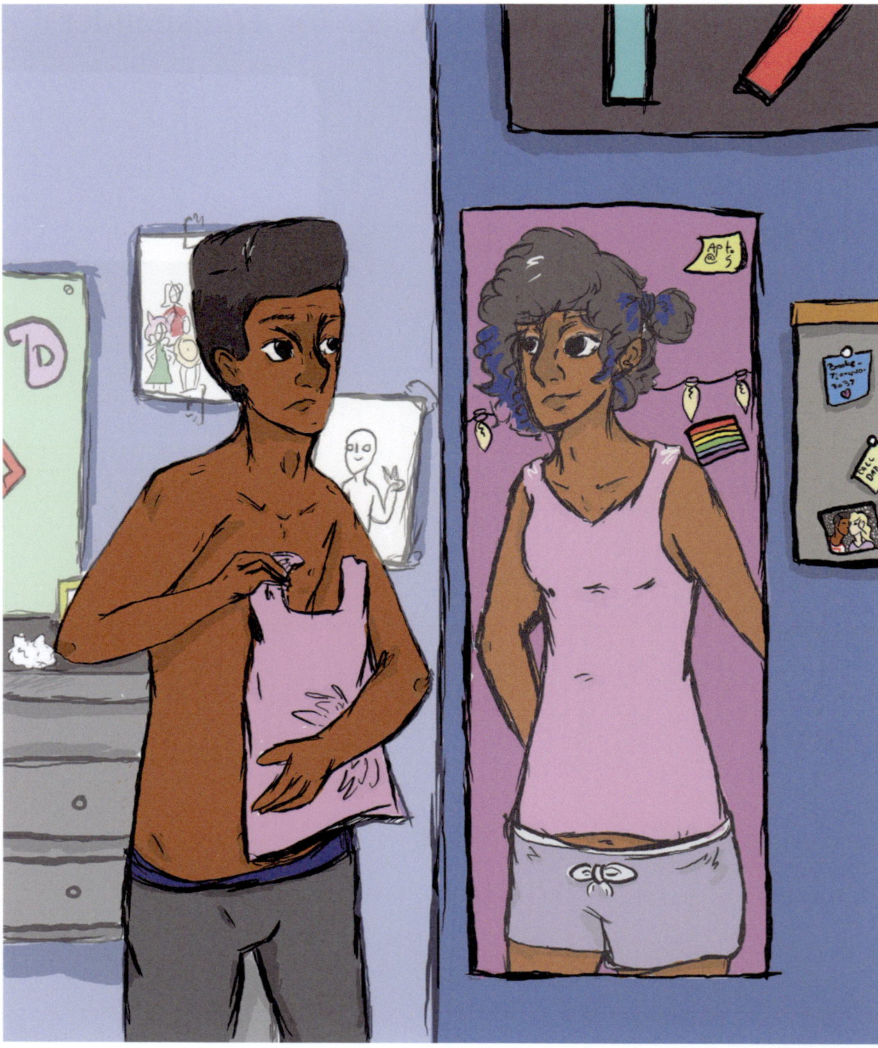

Miles France
Age: 13
Pronouns: He/Him

Aron Janssen • Scott Leibowitz
Editors

Affirmative Mental Health Care for Transgender and Gender Diverse Youth

A Clinical Guide

Springer

Editors
Aron Janssen, MD
Department of Child and Adolescent Psychiatry
The Child Study Center at NYU Langone Medical Center
New York, NY, USA

Scott Leibowitz, MD
Department of Psychiatry
Nationwide Children's Hospital
The Ohio State University College of Medicine
Columbus, OH, USA

ISBN 978-3-319-78306-2 ISBN 978-3-319-78307-9 (eBook)
https://doi.org/10.1007/978-3-319-78307-9

Library of Congress Control Number: 2018941865

Printed on acid-free paper

This Springer imprint is published by the registered company Springer International Publishing AG part of Springer Nature.
The registered company address is: Gewerbestrasse 11, 6330 Cham, Switzerland

Foreword

Families are increasingly reaching out to child and adolescent psychiatrists for support and guidance regarding their gender nonconforming and transgender children. Colleagues in allied professions—social work, psychology, mental and behavioral health care, and medicine—are also seeking consultation regarding clients/patients under their clinical care. The expectation is that child and adolescent psychiatrists have the skills and training to offer comprehensive, expert advice—indeed what is often perceived of as the highest level of clinical expertise in mental health assessment available.

Unfortunately, for many child and adolescent psychiatrists there is huge deficit gap in their education and training regarding working with gender diverse and transgender patients. This is not unusual; indeed, this training gap exists throughout medicine in general, and in all behavioral health education. In order to build collaborative multidisciplinary teams, it is necessary for child and adolescent psychiatrists to grow in competency in working with gender nonconforming children and transgender youth.

Fortunately, Aron Janssen and Scott Leibowitz have provided a casebook that not only educates child and adolescent psychiatrists about diverse gender identity development, but thoroughly integrates this knowledge into the multilayered complexities of mental health assessment and diagnosis. This casebook does not shy away from the complicated questions posed by the interplay of psychopathology, gender identity, and child development; nor does it avoid the ethical challenges presented at the junction where diagnosis and identity development meet within a socio-political landscape.

I am a social worker and family therapist, and I have worked with the transgender community for nearly 30 years. About 15 years ago I published a book called *Transgender Emergence: Therapeutic Guidelines for Working with Gender Variant People and their Families*. The book was the first clinical book to suggest that transgender identity was not a mental illness, a radical idea at the time, and one that labeled me a bit "crazy" by some of my colleagues. Indeed, most of my colleagues at the University did not know what the word transgender meant. The distinction between being a pioneer and lunatic is often a thinner line than we'd like to admit.

Asserting oneself as someone who provides services to this population can mean that one is stepping into the middle of what is both a professional debate about treatment appropriateness and a media debacle.

This book, *Affirmative Mental Health Care for Transgender and Gender Diverse Youth: A Clinical Casebook,* is an invitation to child and adolescent psychiatrists to expand their knowledge base and bring their expertise to a field needing their specific guidance and training. It is not only appropriate for the child and adolescent psychiatrists, but can be beneficial for all mental health professionals across disciplines. Transgender people and their challenges for civil rights have moved into the mainstream, but as professionals we have a long way to go in establishing a clinical community that is responsive and respectful to their complex needs.

In *Transgender Emergence* I stated that I believed that transgender people had been pathologized by the mental health system; indeed, they had been pathologized *just like* "homosexuals" had been decades earlier, and using the same (broken) diagnostic tools and psychological theories of psychogenic mothers, distant fathers, and "normal" development gone awry. People in the helping professions do not like to be accused of causing harm, but we have played a very complex and controversial role in the treatment of sexual and gender minorities—gay, lesbian, bisexual, and transgender people. We have far too often used the power we wield to diagnose and treat pathology that might more clearly be called pathos.

There are very few behavioral health clinicians—regardless of training or degree—that would state today that homosexuality is an illness and should be put back in the diagnostic manuals. The line between mental health diagnoses and political identities is not irrelevant to our clinical work. Throwing off the yoke and stigma of "pathology" facilitated the legal, political, and clinical transformations that could never have been granted a "mentally ill" population. I believe we stand on this precipice again, as allied professionals, in how we think about transgender identity and gender nonconforming expression.

Not that long ago the only models of treatment were reparative models, attempting to fix what we were then called "sissy boys" and "tomboy girls," to make them "normal" through behavior modification. Reparative therapy was the predominant treatment available to clinicians who practiced with this population and preventing adult transgender identity was the primary goal. Suggesting that a child could be completely mentally healthy and transgender was a radical idea, in some measure an oxymoron, an impossibility. That idea has now taken root; it is flourishing in large medical centers and small therapy practices across the western world. We are building a collaborative clinical community to learn together how to bring our skills and compassion together to serve children and youth who stand outside of societally proscribed gender boxes.

Transgender Emergence made another bold claim—that we needed to see trans people as part of families and systems, a part of the beloved community, and that our job as clinicians is to help families embrace and love what we have come to call gender creative children. In the book, *Far from the Tree: Parents, Children, and the Search for Identity,* Andrew Solomon poignantly writes about the complicated experience of having children with whom parents do not share the same identity, and he includes transgender children in his detailed analysis. Although certainly transgender parents can have transgender children, the majority of families that seek the services of professionals have never contemplated having a gender diverse child, and are completely unprepared for the challenges this might evoke. Solomon says, "Parenting abruptly catapults us into a permanent relationship with a stranger." He continues, "Though many of us take pride in how different we are from our parents, we are endlessly sad at how different our children are from us."

The families of gender nonconforming and transgender children and adolescents come seeking the services of professionals because they are scared for their children and sad to find this stranger in their midst, a beloved child who has become a stranger. One of our jobs is to help caregivers recognize this stranger as one of their own, to help them invite their child back into the pack, into the sanctity of their family nest. We need to normalize gender atypical development, and as child and adolescent psychiatrists that is an enormous power, to convey health, and reassure normalcy, to a frightened parent or child. (As I write this, I am reminded of bringing my newly adopted baby to an appointment with a heart specialist, at the suggestion of my son's pediatrician. I was so frightened! After the examination, the good doctor took my hand and looked me in the eye and said, "In my heart of hearts, I think your child is fine." Oh such power we wield, not just in our diagnostics, but in our bedside manner.)

Assuaging parental anguish is not our only job though (after all, if my son's heart was not "okay," our family would have needed even more quality interaction and care). The reality is most children that are brought to professionals, especially those referred to psychiatrists, are having other troubles in addition to those that differences in gender expression has wrought. There is no doubt that being different can invite complicated socio-cultural experiences from school systems, religious communities, and peers. It can evoke rejections, judgment, hostility, and even violence. These can cause as well as increase any psychological challenges one may already be struggling with. In a culture that punishes parents for their children's failings and alienates those that exhibit any difference, what might, within an isolated supportive environment, be a normal developmental process for a child can become a psychiatric maelstrom. It is our job as mental health specialists to sort out these threads: what is normal (even if atypical) gender development, what is psychological distress caused by the complications of difference (oppression, rejection, confusion), and what is psychopathology? And if mental illness is diagnosed, then what is its relationship to the child's gender—etiological, symbiotic (or synergetic), or is it simply a parallel process, like myopia and foot fungus.

Child and adolescent psychiatrists have a very important role to play in the emerging field of trans-health care, yet the gap in training on gender identity and expression is a palpable challenge felt throughout the various disciplines that need to interact as a team in order to provide effective, compassionate, and evidence-based care. As specialists in *both* child development and psychopathology, and experts in *both* interpersonal family relationships and human physiology, child and adolescent psychiatrists bring a set of skills to the table that are essential to our work with transgender children and youth. Effective care that promotes wellness for trans youth requires that child and adolescent psychiatrists also understand that gender diversity as an isolated construct does not implicitly assume pathology, yet gender dysphoria can cause mental health challenges and significantly impact the approach to assessment, diagnostic clarity, and management of other mental health conditions.

This book, *Affirmative Mental Health Care for Transgender and Gender Diverse Youth: A Clinical Casebook,* is a broad overview of the type of cases that might present in treatment, including those presenting with complex psychiatric issues including depression, anxiety, ADHD, and psychotic disorders. Additionally, there are chapters addressing the interface between transgender identity and other human differences which can impact diagnoses and identity development including disorders/differences in sex development and autism. Attention is given to those presenting with nonbinary identities and cultural/linguistic/ethnic issues which can influence treatment. Highlighted throughout are careful steps towards comprehensive and collaborative interdisciplinary assessment processes.

Generally, when a child or youth is being referred to a psychiatrist there are multiple overlapping issues that need to be sorted through diagnostically. Understanding why the child is being referred to the psychiatrist is important. Is the child articulating a transgender identity and are the parents confused or skeptical and wanting an expert opinion? Is the child experiencing mental health struggles like anxiety or depression, and referred by another mental health provider who is seeking psychopharmacological intervention as adjunctive to their treatment? Is the youth presenting with cognitive or psychiatric symptoms that confound the diagnostic process requiring a more specialized gender-informed psychiatric assessment with the intention of clarifying treatment goals that appropriately address the underlying root issues? Perhaps the timing of starting a social or medical transition requires the expertise of a psychiatrist as part of the multidisciplinary team due to the complexity of psychological, familial, or medical complications of the case?

The consulting child and adolescent psychiatrist brings particular skillsets to the assessment process, in terms of recognizing the complexity of interpersonal relationships within the family when gender dysphoria and adolescent rebellion cross paths. They bring holistic biopsychosocial skills to assess cognitive, psychiatric, and developmental processes in maturing children and youth. They can bring a high level of knowledge and sophistication regarding physiology, brain development, and other medical health-related issues and how those can influence human development. However, these skillsets are only useful within an affirmative gender-informed treatment model, one that far too few child and adolescent psychiatrists have been trained to utilize.

If the psychiatrist believes that there is only a binary of male/female gender expression, and pathologizes all gender atypical behavior, nonbinary identities, or transgender experience, then a healthy child will be viewed as mentally ill for what are normative developmental processes. If a psychiatrist thinks that gender atypical behavior is always etiologically related to mental health issues that may be present (i.e., the child is saying they are transgender just because they are also autistic; the youth identifies as nonbinary because they have PTSD from a gang rape), then they are not only pathologizing the child, but are perhaps recommending the withholding of necessary medical treatments for their gender authenticity. Sorting out the normative challenges of being a child or adolescent who is gender divergent from societal expectations from other complex mental health challenges can only begin from an affirmative stance that supports gender diversity and transgender identity.

However, gender-informed affirmative care also means that a psychiatrist brings the breadth of their assessment skill to clinical processes and recognizes that gender can sometimes be a symptom of mental health struggles. The timing of treatments—gender treatments and psychopharmacological treatments for mental health issues—should be carefully thought out so they support normative development and ease gender dysphoria.

In the last decade, we have witnessed transgender people moving from the margins of society onto the center stage of civil rights struggles. On the shoulders of a feminist movement that challenged rigid gender role stereotypes, and a lesbian and gay community that celebrated the right to authenticity, transgender people have emerged from the shadows and are demanding their right to fully live their lives. Thirty years ago, Gayle Rubin said that "Sexualities keep marching out of the Diagnostic and Statistical Manual and on to the pages of social history," and indeed we see this march from the pathologization of sexual and gender minorities to integration of LGBT people within the wider human society.

Without these large socio-political movements, young children would not likely have found a way to voice cross-gender feelings to their parents, and transgender teens would have kept their thoughts buried, trying to fit into the society as best they could. As therapists, we can imagine the psychological challenges that come from suppressing core parts of one's identity, manifesting in mental health and behavioral struggles. There is nothing new about gender diversity or gender dysphoria for children and youth; indeed these children have been on our caseloads for years. What is new is that children and youth are expressing their feelings and experiences now within social-cultural environments and families that are responding in affirming ways. They are seeking out the services of professionals who must become experts in this newly emerging field, one which invites us to re-examine developmental theories embedded in our previous training.

Political movements for liberation have, once again, challenged therapeutic communities to review the legacies of our predecessors. We are called upon to question our views of "normal" human development and of what we have learned about the formation of sex and gender identities. Through the development of gender-affirmative care we are invited to become leaders in re-defining mental health and wellness.

Although we are still perhaps pioneers navigating a new landscape, we are not without a map. Scott Leibowitz, Aron Janssen, and their collaborators in this casebook have articulated guidelines, with clear directions—and they have done so using the best tool possible—case assessment. Everyone knows the experience of reading textbooks on theory, and the frustration of applicability to the actual humans in our office. These case analyses give the reader the opportunity to see how colleagues with expertise assess complex information and develop treatment plans that are embedded in both solid psychiatric knowledge and gender-affirmative care. I hope that child and adolescent psychiatrists who are holding this book in your hands understand that it is a gift that can open up a door that will change how you see—not just gender creative and transgender children and adolescents—but every child and adolescent in your care.

Albany, NY, USA Arlene Lev, LCSW-R, CASAC, CST

Preface

Early in our training, we each distinctly recall those situations where we encountered youth presenting to crisis services because, for one reason or another, they could not come to terms with their gender identity: whether it was the adolescent patient who was admitted to the inpatient psychiatric unit after an overdose in the context of struggling to accept her gender identity or the ten year old in the emergency room saying he did not want to live because the other children teased him that day for choosing the pink frame in art class. At the time, nobody on the unit or emergency room had a sense of how to best address the gender component of who they were. There were no clinical guidelines or casebooks that we could find to help better understand their needs and how to tailor our approach. For us, that sense of inefficacy and ignorance led us both to want to learn as much as possible to be able to provide competent care and to better advocate for the needs of our gender diverse patients. At that time, it was rare to have a transgender adolescent on the inpatient unit. In the emergency room, the fact that a child would be bullied due to innate aspects of their gender expression would be overlooked when the clinician would formulate what was happening in that situation. Today, it is much more common for clinicians to encounter transgender and gender diverse youth across all ages and all types of clinical practices. Ten years ago there were only a handful of multidisciplinary gender clinics in the United States and now there are over 50. Yet somehow there is still a woeful lack of training on working with these youth.

It is in responding to this lack of training, and in particular, the unmet mental health needs of transgender and gender diverse youth that this book has been written. What lies in the chapters ahead is content that will improve your *gender competence*, that is, your ability to formulate *all* of your patients' needs, recognizing that every child, adolescent, and person has a gender identity, gender expression, and sexual orientation. And for some, it plays a role in the clinical presentation in the moment, while for others it does not, and we must be cognizant of the fact that these phenomena are distinct from one another, yet also interrelated. For those youth who are gender diverse and/or transgender, it is a population that is increasingly growing within the clinical world and all too often mental health clinicians do not feel equipped to manage the issues that are coming up in their practices.

Some may ask why clinicians are seeing so many more transgender youth. Are there simply more transgender youth? Has increased visibility of transgender youth and adults in the media led to more youth being able to define an experience that previous youth had no ability to name? Has society shifted away from a binary conceptualization of gender and more towards thinking about gender along a spectrum? Regardless of the reason, we need to be able to define best practices and adhere to the current standards of care while providing effective mental health treatment. The gap in training needs to be closed. These youth and families need our help and they need compassionate and evidence-based care. The stigma and mental health disparities are alarming and lives are at stake. Prompt treatment is needed and clinicians need to be able to recognize when gender affirming interventions are indicated.

Our casebook has several aims for the child and adolescent psychiatrist and other mental health professionals looking to improve their skillset when working with these youth. The first three chapters set the stage and provide the reader with practical information about assessment, psychological interventions, and medical/surgical interventions used with the population, respectively. The remaining ten chapters are case chapters that utilize cases to illustrate overarching points. In these chapters, readers are provided with broad questions that are applicable in clinical practice in the beginning of the chapter. The cases themselves, written by our expert clinicians in the field, are used to answer the questions laid out in the beginning of each chapter. At the end of each chapter, clinical take-home messages are provided for the reader.

Each of the case chapters focuses on a particular co-occurring condition or theme. The first three of these case chapters give the reader an overview of cases where the main central theme is not rooted in psychopathology but rather about some other element that might be seen in clinical practice. These three case chapters delve into youth with complex family dynamics, youth declaring a nonbinary gender identity, and a youth born with a difference/disorder of sex development.

The remaining case chapters each focus on a specific co-occurring psychiatric condition. You will notice our use of the term *co-occurring* instead of *co-morbid.* This is intentional as we approach gender diversity itself as a nonpathological entity. In these case chapters that focus on a co-occurring psychiatric condition, the authors first provide a brief review of the scientific literature specific to the various co-occurring psychopathologies. They then address the specific clinical needs and interventions for children and adolescents experiencing gender-related concerns in the context of co-occurring psychopathology. In this way, the authors begin to tease apart, in a case-by-case way, how to differentiate between the types of psychopathologies and how best to intervene. While there are numerous psychopathologies that exist in actual clinical practice, we focus on some of the main diagnoses that present more frequently: anxiety, trauma, depression/suicidal ideation, autism, and attention deficit hyperactivity disorder, and one of the chapters delves into cases where the youth present with complex multiple psychopathologies. While our book does not (and cannot) include every single type of co-occurring psychopathology that is represented in the DSM, we hope that the principles addressed in the cases that we do present can be applied to other situations.

Our book has an esteemed group of authors that represent multiple disciplines: psychology, social work, pediatric endocrinology, pediatric urology, advanced psychiatric nurse practitioners, and child and adolescent psychiatrists. All of the authors have extensive experience working with transgender and gender diverse youth. The case chapters include scenarios that approach the full developmental spectrum from prepubertal children to older adolescents, and accordingly address the gender affirming interventions that fit with each age group. There is also ethnic, racial, and cultural diversity in the clinical cases described, as intersectionality is an important theme that comes up in the care of these youth and we firmly believe that the clinician should be aware of the full biopsychosocial picture of the youth and families when developing treatment alliances and guiding families through decision making. Some of the case chapters have juxtaposing cases where one case presents a clearer picture while the other is more complex, therefore helping the mental health professional learn to appreciate which of the presenting factors to prioritize in treatment, both in the beginning of treatment and as the treatment progresses.

This casebook is the first of its kind. We believe that clinicians across all mental health disciplines will find it useful, not just child and adolescent psychiatrists. If it has made its way to your hands, then clearly this is a subject that you are hoping to learn more about. With each chapter being independent from one another, we hope you will find it user friendly to read and that it will be a resource to you when helping this vulnerable group of children and families. We hope you find this casebook as rewarding to read as we did to compile, edit, and write.

New York, NY, USA Aron Janssen, MD
Columbus, OH, USA Scott Leibowitz, MD

Contents

Contributors

Eric N. Boyum, MD Department of Child and Adolescent Psychiatry, University of Iowa Stead Family Children's Hospital, Iowa City, IA, USA

Samantha M. Busa, PsyD Department of Child and Adolescent Psychiatry, Hassenfeld Children's Hospital at NYU Langone, New York, NY, USA

David Call, MD Division of Psychiatry and Behavioral Sciences, Children's National Health System, Washington, DC, USA

Diane Chen, PhD Division of Adolescent Medicine, Department of Child and Adolescent Psychiatry, Ann and Robert H. Lurie Children's Hospital of Chicago, Chicago, IL, USA

Department of Psychiatry and Behavioral Sciences, Northwestern University Feinberg School of Medicine, Chicago, IL, USA

Department of Pediatrics, Northwestern University Feinberg School of Medicine, Chicago, IL, USA

Peter Daniolos, MD Department of Child and Adolescent Psychiatry, University of Iowa Stead Family Children's Hospital, Iowa City, IA, USA

Laura Edwards-Leeper, PhD School of Graduate Psychology, Pacific University, Hillsboro, OR, USA

Courtney A. Finlayson, MD Department of Pediatrics, Northwestern University Feinberg School of Medicine, Chicago, IL, USA

Division of Endocrinology, Northwestern University Feinberg School of Medicine, Chicago, IL, USA

Department of Pediatrics, Ann and Robert H. Lurie Children's Hospital of Chicago, Chicago, IL, USA

Shane W. Gahn, MS, APRN-CNP Department of Psychiatry, Nationwide Children's Hospital, THRIVE: Gender and Sex Development, Columbus, OH, USA

Marco A. Hidalgo, PhD Division of Adolescent and Young Adult Medicine, Center for Transyouth Health and Development, Children's Hospital Los Angeles, Keck School of Medicine of the University of Southern California, Los Angeles, CA, USA

Rebecca Hopkinson, MD Department of Psychiatry and Behavioral Sciences, Seattle Children's Hospital, University of Washington, Seattle, WA, USA

Brandon S. Ito, MD, MPH Department of Psychiatry, UCLA Semel Institute for Neuroscience and Human Behavior, Los Angeles, CA, USA

Aron Janssen, MD Department of Child and Adolescent Psychiatry, NYU Langone Health, NYU Child Study Center, New York, NY, USA

Emilie K. Johnson, MD, MPH Division of Urology, Ann and Robert H. Lurie Children's Hospital of Chicago, Chicago, IL, USA

Departments of Urology and Surgery, Center for Healthcare Studies, Northwestern Feinberg School of Medicine, Chicago, IL, USA

Elizabeth Leeth, MS, CGC Departments of Pathology and Pediatrics, Ann and Robert H. Lurie Children's Hospital of Chicago, Chicago, IL, USA

Scott Leibowitz, MD Department of Psychiatry, THRIVE Gender and Sex Development Program, Nationwide Children's Hospital, Columbus, OH, USA

Department of Psychiatry, The Ohio State University College of Medicine, Columbus, OH, USA

Melissa MacNish, MA, LMHC Licensed Mental Health, SAYFTEE, LLC, Jamaica Plain, MA, USA

Nathaniel G. Sharon, MD Division of Child and Adolescent Psychiatry, Department of Psychiatry and Behavioral Sciences, University of New Mexico, Albuquerque, NM, USA

Valerie Tobin, MS, APN, PMHCNS-BC Behavioral Health Services, Howard Brown Health, Chicago, IL, USA

Robert Wood Johnson Future of Nursing Scholar, Rush University College of Nursing, Chicago, IL, USA

Elizabeth B. Yerkes, MD Department of Urology, Ann and Robert H. Lurie Children's Hospital of Chicago, Chicago, IL, USA

Departments of Urology and Surgery, Center for Healthcare Studies, Northwestern Feinberg School of Medicine, Chicago, IL, USA

Chapter 1
Affirming and Gender-Informed Assessment of Gender Diverse and/or Transgender Youth Across Development

Scott Leibowitz and Aron Janssen

Introduction

Youth across development are presenting with gender identity concerns to mental health professionals with increasing prevalence over the past decade. Families may present for a variety of reasons and with a variety of chief complaints. The child and adolescent psychiatrist (CAP) or mental health provider (MHP) may play a crucial role in assisting these youth and families, many of whom are struggling for answers and a direction. Within the field of behavioral health, psychiatrists, psychologists, social workers, allied health professionals, and other mental health counselors have been through training programs that vary in the degree to which they have been trained and/or educated on gender development, family dynamics, psychodiagnostics, and psychopathology. Expertise in all domains is crucial when making diagnostic, formulation, and treatment decisions in concert with youth and their families.

Youth presenting with gender issues encompass a larger umbrella group under which the youth specifically meeting criteria for gender dysphoria (GD) of either childhood or adolescence, which have two distinct criteria sets, may fall [1]. Prior to the DSM-5, the term gender dysphoria was known exclusively as a phenomenon, not a diagnosis with criteria. Henceforth, when referring to the diagnostic classification, we will use the acronym GD, and when referring to the phenomenon, we will use the lowercase version, gender dysphoria.

S. Leibowitz, MD (✉)
Department of Psychiatry, THRIVE Gender and Sex Development Program, Nationwide Children's Hospital, Columbus, OH, USA

Department of Psychiatry, The Ohio State University College of Medicine, Columbus, OH, USA

A. Janssen, MD
Department of Child and Adolescent Psychiatry, NYU Langone Health, NYU Child Study Center, New York, NY, USA

A. Janssen, S. Leibowitz (eds.), *Affirmative Mental Health Care for Transgender and Gender Diverse Youth*, https://doi.org/10.1007/978-3-319-78307-9_1

Consensus regarding aspects of the assessment of youth with gender dysphoria has not yet been reached across disciplines. Empirical data in this field lacks, mostly due to the nascence of the field. In 2007 there was only one formal multidisciplinary gender clinic in an academic pediatric children's hospital, and by 2014 it had grown to more than 40 [2], with even more clinics having emerged since then. Therefore, it is important we state up front that this assessment chapter is based on the *clinical experience of the authors* from their perspective as child and adolescent psychiatrists and not entirely rooted in empirically validated data. To the best extent we can, we will point out whether or not there is scientific backing regarding a description of the assessment approach.

Framing the Gender-Informed Assessment

There is wide variation among the youth in terms of how they present their gender, what types of interventions they seek, how their families think about gender, and whether or not they have a co-occurring psychological or psychiatric issue. Some youth may specifically be seeking interventions that will affect their physical bodies – pubertal suppression, sex hormones, and/or surgeries. In some situations, other physicians and/or therapists may be referring the youth to a CAP or MHP with the same question: *Is it clinically appropriate to move forward with sought after interventions that may or may not lead to irreversible changes on the youth's body?*

Contextualizing the aims of the assessment is important, as the purpose or reason why the youth and/or family winds up in the CAP or MHP's office can vary. The MHP may sometimes be asked to assess for diagnostic clarity with the purpose of developing a biopsychosocial formulation and gender-informed treatment plan. Other times, the provider may be asked to assess for the appropriateness of a specific gender-affirming medical intervention based on specific criteria or about the potential impact of gender-affirming medical interventions on independent mental health concerns. Specifically for the CAP, a referring provider may want a targeted assessment for appropriateness of psychopharmacological interventions or to understand how hormones and surgery may impact the psychiatric medications already prescribed. Clarifying the assessment aims in the beginning of treatment, sometimes prior to meeting the child and family, can be useful so that the frame of the assessment can be determined up front. It is also important to note that while a referring provider or a particular family may be presenting to the CAP or MHP with specific intentions and/or ideas about timing, the assessment process may reveal other concerns that may also benefit from intervention.

For example, a CAP may be meeting a family expecting to begin psychopharmacological interventions, yet they may be shortly starting gender-affirming hormone treatment within a very short time frame. Starting two interventions in close proximity may pose challenges in terms of being able to assess treatment response to a particular intervention. In this scenario, the CAP needs to determine the underlying cause of the presenting complaint and therefore be able to work collaboratively with the youth, their family, and referring providers to thoroughly understand the potential risks and benefits of each decision. For one youth, this might mean initiating a psychopharmacological intervention and therefore delaying the gender-affirming hormone treatment. For another youth, it might mean starting the gender-affirming hormone treatment, determining response, and reassessing need for a psychopharmacological intervention in the future depending on what is happening then. Both scenarios may lead to disappointment in the family and/or youth since the frame of the assessment was presumed before the assessment took place. Laying the groundwork beforehand by establishing the frame rooted in a communicative and collaborative model with other providers can mitigate these potential disappointments.

Another scenario may be that the CAP or MHP is tasked with doing an assessment for "hormone readiness" in an adolescent who another medical provider may have determined meets diagnostic criteria for GD. That provider may have referred the family to the CAP or MHP under the premise that this is a "readiness assessment," which may influence the youth and family about what they feel the scope of the assessment should be. In a situation such as this, it may be possible that in doing the assessment, it may become unclear whether the adolescent does in fact meet criteria for GD. The adolescent and family may have approached the appointment with unfair expectations and may feel disappointed should the frame of the assessment shift once it is underway.

To that end, the concept of the *affirmative gender-informed* assessment may be useful to explain before starting with the family. The goal of the affirmative gender-informed assessment is to work collaboratively with the young person, their family, and their other providers to provide support and care, allowing room for the young person to explore their identity in a non-pathologizing way and supporting interventions to maximize long-term wellness and functioning. The premise is that there is no initial agenda other than to be open-ended in the exploration of diagnostic and treatment possibilities, all while appreciating the fact that gender diversity does not imply psychopathology, obtaining a diagnosis of GD may or may not be accurate after only a few appointments (depending on the child or adolescent), and that a holistic biopsychosocial formulation (as one would do with any youth) helps provide important clarity to guide the formulation and treatment recommendations. Therefore, staying clear from terms such as *readiness assessment* (which implies the person is on a path toward a particular treatment but may or may not be ready for it), *gender assessment* (which implies that the provider is telling the family what the child or adolescent's gender is), or *psychopharmacological assessment* (which implies medications are indicated) may be useful in reducing iatrogenic disappointment when expectations are not met.

Terminology

Terminology that describes domains of gender and sexuality is important to deconstruct for any provider working with children and adolescents. Youth may often use terms to describe their identity, yet this does not always cohere with the formal nomenclature used to make a clinical classification according to the DSM-5. Clarifying how a youth uses a certain term is important for the CAP or MHP considering different youth may use terms in different ways. To that end, Table 1.1 illustrates the definitions that are commonly recognized in the field from a professional standpoint. They represent a compilation of terms described in the American Academy of Child and Adolescent Psychiatry *Practice Parameter on Gay, Lesbian or Bisexual Sexual Orientation, Gender Nonconformity, and Gender Discordance in Children and Adolescents* [3, pp. 5–6] and the Endocrine Society's *Endocrine Treatment of Gender-Dysphoric/Gender-Incongruent Persons: An Endocrine Society Clinical Practice Guideline* [4, p. 7].

Table 1.1 Relevant terminology

Assigned sex at birth (also referred to as birth-assigned sex, birth-assigned males, or birth-assigned females): This refers to the sex that is given to an infant at birth and is usually based on genital anatomy
Cisgender: This is the antonym for transgender, describing an alignment between gender identity and assigned sex at birth
Gender-affirming (hormone) treatment (also cross-sex hormones, cross-gender hormones): This refers to the provision of sex hormones (testosterone or estrogen) to individuals with gender dysphoria to closer align secondary sex characteristics with the person's experienced gender identity
Gender dysphoria: This is the distress and unease experienced if gender identity and designated gender are not completely congruent. In 2013, the American Psychiatric Association released the fifth edition of the DSM-5, which replaced "gender identity disorder" with "gender dysphoria" and changed the criteria for diagnosis, which we will use the acronym GD henceforth when referring to the clinical classification
Gender expression (or gender role behavior): This refers to external manifestations of gender, expressed through one's name, pronouns, mannerisms, clothing, haircut, behavior, voice, or body characteristics
Gender fluid: This is typically used to refer to changes in gender identity *or* expression over time, depending on how the individual uses the term
Gender identity/experienced gender (also referred to as "affirmed gender"): This refers to one's internal, deeply held sense of gender. For transgender people, their gender identity does not match their assigned sex at birth. For cisgender people, their gender identity does match their assigned sex at birth. Unlike gender expression (see below), gender identity is not visible to others. Gender identity usually develops by age 3 and remains stable over the lifetime; however, for a small number of individuals, it can change later in life
Gender incongruence (also referred to as gender discordance): This is an umbrella term used when the gender identity and/or gender expression differs from what is typically associated with the assigned sex at birth which usually designates gender. Gender incongruence is also the proposed name of the gender identity-related diagnoses in ICD-11. Not all individuals with gender incongruence have gender dysphoria or seek treatment
Gender nonbinary: This refers to individuals who do not identify as one of the binary male or female genders but potentially aspects of both or neither

Gender nonconforming (also referred to as gender diverse, gender variant, gender expansive, gender creative): This refers to variation from norms in gender role behavior that is typical for a particular age or developmental stage. Not all individuals who are gender nonconforming or gender diverse would identify as transgender or meet criteria for GD
Gender reassignment: This refers to the treatment procedure for those who want to adapt their bodies to the experienced gender by means of hormones and/or surgery. This is also called gender-confirming or gender-affirming treatment
Gender reassignment surgery (gender-confirming/gender-affirming surgery, previously known as sex reassignment surgery): These terms refer only to the surgical component of gender reassignment
Gender role: This refers to behaviors, attitudes, and personality traits that a society (in a given culture and historical period) designates as masculine or feminine and/or that society associates with or considers typical of the social role of men or women
Sex: This refers to attributes that characterize biological maleness or femaleness. The best known attributes include the sex-determining genes, the sex chromosomes, the H-Y antigen, the gonads, sex hormones, internal and external genitalia, and secondary sex characteristics
Sexual orientation: This term describes an individual's enduring physical and emotional attraction to another person. Gender identity and sexual orientation are not the same. Irrespective of their gender identity, transgender people may be attracted to women (gynephilic), attracted to men (androphilic), bisexual, asexual, or queer
Transgender: This is an umbrella term for people whose gender identity and/or gender expression differs from what is typically associated with their sex designated at birth. Not all transgender individuals seek treatment
Transgender male (also trans man, female to male, transgender male): This refers to individuals assigned female at birth but who identify and live as men
Transgender woman (also trans woman, male to female, transgender female): This refers to individuals assigned male at birth but who identify and live as women
Transition: This refers to the process during which transgender persons change their physical, social, and/or legal characteristics consistent with the affirmed gender identity. Prepubertal children may choose to transition socially. Transsexual: This is an older term that originated in the medical and psychological communities to refer to individuals who have permanently transitioned through medical interventions or desired to do so

Role of the Mental Health Provider in Gender-Informed Assessment

Across all stages of development, the American Academy of Child and Adolescent Psychiatry *Practice Parameter on Gay, Lesbian or Bisexual Sexual Orientation, Gender Nonconformity, and Gender Discordance in Children and Adolescents* is clear in Principle 1 that a "comprehensive diagnostic evaluation should include an age-appropriate assessment of psychosexual development for all youths" [3, p. 14]. The interventions that may be clinically indicated depend on the stage of development and are discussed further in Chaps. 2 and 3 of this casebook.

However, as far as whether or not an evaluation by a CAP or MHP is recommended prior to the initiation of medical interventions (including GnRH analogs and sex hormones) for an adolescent with GD, other guidelines point to the clinical utility of comprehensive assessment. The Endocrine Society Guidelines [4] and

World Professional Association of Transgender Health, Standards of Care 7th edition [5] both recommend that a biopsychosocial assessment of youth is performed prior to the initiation of any medical treatments for adolescents with gender dysphoria.

Per the Endocrine Society Guidelines, a mental health provider diagnosing GD in children and adolescents should meet the following criteria: (1) training in child and adolescent developmental psychology and psychopathology, (2) competence in using the DSM and/or ICD for diagnostic purposes, (3) the ability to make a distinction between GD/gender incongruence and conditions that have similar features (e.g., body dysmorphic disorder), (4) training in diagnosing psychiatric conditions, (5) the ability to undertake or refer for appropriate treatment, (6) the ability to psychosocially assess the person's understanding and social conditions that can impact gender-affirming hormone therapy, (7) a practice of regularly attending relevant professional meetings, and (8) knowledge of the criteria for puberty blocking and gender-affirming hormone treatment in adolescents. The Endocrine Society Guidelines further stipulate that the presence of the diagnostic criteria for GD is necessary before initiating pubertal suppression, gender-affirming hormones, and/or potential surgical interventions [4].

Gaps in knowledge on the assessment and treatment of gender dysphoria in childhood and adolescence invariably exist given that not all child and adolescent psychiatry training programs include this component of training into their curriculum. It is for that reason that a casebook such as this exists – to further educate providers across all points in their career, whether they have access to a multidisciplinary team of providers or not.

Diagnostic Criteria

The DSM-5 lists gender dysphoria as a diagnostic entity with two subtypes, one for children and another for adolescents/adults. Tables 1.2 and 1.3 list the separate criteria for both classifications. It is important to note that not all children or adolescents that may identify as something other than cisgender will experience distress or dysfunction as a result of their identity, particularly when in supportive environments. In this case, a child may be both transgender and yet not meet diagnostic criteria for GD. As such, ensuring that a child or adolescent meets criteria for GD may or may not be simple, but it is useful in developing a treatment plan that is both identity affirming and effective.

It is important to note that *on the surface*, meeting the criteria for GD may seem straightforward. However, in many situations as the biopsychosocial assessment provides additional clarity to the overarching psychological and psychiatric picture of the child, adolescent, and family, it may become clear that additional time beyond that what is designated for the assessment will be useful in helping further tease apart the gender-related concerns that are being brought to the MHP or CAP initially. Therefore, as a diagnostician would do in any other situation where a

Table 1.2 DSM-5 criteria for gender dysphoria in children[a]

A. A marked incongruence between one's experience/expressed gender and natal gender of at least 6 months in duration, as manifested by at least six of the following eight indicators, at least one of which must be criterion A1: 1. A strong desire to be of the other gender or an insistence that one is the other gender (or some alternative gender different from one's assigned gender) 2. In boys (assigned gender), a strong preference for cross-dressing or simulating female attire; or in girls (assigned gender), a strong preference for wearing only typical masculine clothing and a strong resistance to wearing of typical feminine clothing 3. A strong preference for cross-gender roles in make-believe play or fantasy play 4. A strong preference for toys, games, or activities stereotypically used or engaged in by the other gender 5. A strong preference for the playmates of the other gender 6. In boys (assigned gender), a strong rejection of typically masculine toys, games, and activities and a strong avoidance of rough-and-tumble play; or in girls (assigned gender), a strong rejection of typically feminine toys, games, and activities 7. A strong dislike of one's anatomy 8. A strong desire for the primary and/or secondary sex characteristics that match one's experienced gender
B. The condition is associated with clinically significant distress or impairment in social, school, or other important areas of functioning

[a]APA 2013 [1]

Table 1.3 DSM-5 criteria for gender dysphoria in adolescents and adults[a]

A. A marked incongruence between one's experience/expressed gender and natal gender of at least 6 months in duration, as manifested by at least two of the following: 1. A marked incongruence between one's experienced/expressed gender and primary and/or secondary sex characteristics (or in young adolescents, the anticipated secondary sex characteristics) 2. A strong desire to be rid of one's primary and/or secondary sex characteristics because of a marked incongruence with one's experienced/expressed gender (or in young adolescents, a desire to prevent the development of the anticipated secondary sex characteristics) 3. A strong desire for the primary and/or secondary sex characteristics of the other gender 4. A strong desire to be of the other gender (or some alternative gender different from one's designated gender) 5. A strong desire to be treated as the other gender (or some alternative gender different from one's designated gender) 6. A strong conviction that one has the typical feelings and reactions of the other gender (or some alternative gender different from one's designated gender)
B. The condition is associated with clinically significant distress or impairment in social, occupational, or other important areas of functioning
Specify if: 1. The condition exists with a disorder of sex development 2. The condition is posttransitional, in that the individual has transitioned to full-time living in the desired gender (with or without legalization of gender change) and has undergone (or is preparing to have) at least one sex-related medical procedure or treatment regimen – namely, regular sex hormone treatment or gender reassignment surgery confirming the desired gender (e.g., penectomy, vaginoplasty in natal males; mastectomy or phalloplasty in natal females)

[a]APA 2013 [1]

diagnosis is not clear, considering the diagnosis as *provisional* and identifying treatment goals that address ways to establish diagnostic certainty are important by the end of the specified assessment period.

Psychopathology in Youth Presenting with Gender-Related Concerns

The presence of psychopathology among youth with gender-related concerns is controversial in that most of the studies of psychiatric functioning of youth with gender identity concerns are culled from the clinically referred population. Among this group, across the board, anxiety is the most frequent co-occurring complaint, with approximately 20–30% of individuals presenting to a gender clinic meeting DSM criteria for an anxiety disorder. Disruptive behavior disorders, including ADHD, were the next most common followed by mood disorders and autism spectrum disorders [6]. The case chapters (Chaps. 4–13) will review these common co-occurrences and what is and is not known. Notably, while these numbers are significantly higher than in the general population, they are actually lower than the number of co-occurrences of psychiatric diagnoses when compared to a non-GD clinic referred population. Stated in another way, a child presenting with ADHD or anxiety is more likely to have a co-occurring psychiatric diagnosis than a child presenting with gender dysphoria, and the most common co-occurring psychopathology for a child with gender dysphoria is no co-occurring psychopathology at all.

And yet children with gender-related concerns do have significantly increased co-occurring psychopathology than the general population. These concerns can lead to a significant decline in functioning, which may cloud the diagnostic process and decision-making about gender-affirming interventions much more difficult. The challenge is to not lose sight of the impact of gender-related concerns on overall mental wellness and also to not lose sight of the impact of co-occurring psychopathologies on both the presentation of gender-related concerns and the preparedness for interventions.

In clinical work, we see three main types of psychopathology in youth presenting with gender identity concerns. The first is psychopathology secondary to the experience of stigma and discrimination. The second is psychopathology resultant from the gender dysphoria itself. The third is psychopathology that is independent of the gender identity concerns that nevertheless may influence how an individual experiences and expresses their gender.

In considering the presence of psychopathology in individuals presenting with gender identity concerns, it is important first to understand the concept of minority stress theory. Minority stress theory describes the negative impact to medical and mental health as a result of chronically high stress experienced by members of stigmatized minority groups [7, 8]. Historically (and presently), transgender individuals have faced family rejection, high rates of homelessness and victimization and trauma, few opportunities for gainful employment, and significant interpersonal discrimination [9]. Transgender individuals are more likely to receive inadequate health care and historically have been seen by mental health professionals as inherently mentally ill. As a result, particularly in regard to mental health concerns, individuals with negative experiences would be expected to avoid care, even when it could be beneficial.

Prior to adulthood, children and adolescents often learn that their experience of their gender is something that must be hidden and is something about which to be ashamed. As individuals come to terms with their gender identity, they are often able to point to these times in their lives when they felt their true selves recede away and felt compelled to hide their identity from those from which they needed the most support.

Taken together, the felt effects of overt and covert discrimination and bias paired with the long-term effects of internalized transphobia, we would expect that individuals with GD, just as those from any other stigmatized minority group, would be more likely to experience psychopathology than those without GD. This is in fact what studies of youth with gender dysphoria presenting for treatment have shown. There are significantly higher rates of anxiety, depression, self-harm, and suicide attempts. Interestingly, earlier studies have consistently shown more co-occurring psychopathology than more recent studies, which is what one may expect when individuals are exposed to less stigmatization and more affirmation.

Gender dysphoria itself can also lead to co-occurring psychopathology. For example, many individuals describe a fearfulness of being singled out as a part of the social transition process, which may lead to social avoidance, withdrawal, and anxiety. Many individuals feel hopeless, particularly when in a family that is not supportive of their identity, which can lead to depression, self-harm, and suicide attempts. The reality of increased rates of victimization may lead to panic attacks, and children without access to puberty blockers may stop eating in order to halt the progress of puberty and the feared changes of the body. The secondary effects of GD are as unique as the individuals that experience them and will be reviewed in the subsequent cases. For these secondary effects, we would expect that treating the GD would alleviate or even completely eliminate the presence of these co-occurring psychopathologies.

And finally, gender-related concerns know no social class, geography, race, class, or any other grouping one could imagine. Individuals experiencing their gender identity as something other than aligning completely with their sex assigned at birth have always existed, and we would not expect these individuals to be spared from psychopathology that is independent from the incongruence they experience. As such, it is important to consider the role that potential underlying psychopathology may have on gender-related concerns. Are the gender-related concerns related to the psychopathology itself? For example, does a patient experience distress in their gender only during times of acute mania that resolves with the resolution of the mood symptoms? Is the psychopathology independent of the gender-related concerns but may nevertheless impact one's preparedness for interventions? Historically, individuals with poorly controlled psychopathology have been barred access from transition-related care, but recent case reports point to even individuals with chronic psychotic conditions and GD benefit from treating both conditions concurrently.

Structure of the Assessment

Length

Balancing the demand for patient volume, need to promptly develop a treatment plan for time-dependent interventions, and need to be comprehensive in understanding the many factors that could influence accurately capturing a definitive GD diagnosis requires developing an assessment model that is both timely and thorough. Multiple visits over time within the assessment phase itself may be useful or necessary depending on the length of time that the provider has with the family initially, how much collateral information they have been provided in advance, and how straightforward the clinical picture may be. Some youth and families may respond to the interactions themselves with the provider once a therapeutic alliance is established and myths about the provider's intentions are dispelled vis-à-vis gender identity concerns. For example, the provider who eliminates fears about having a particular agenda other than a desire for the youth to flourish emotionally, psychologically, intellectually, and socially may allow all members of a family to feel more able to disclose authentic feelings about the child or adolescent, whether all together or separate. Sometimes allowing the youth and families time in between assessment appointments helps to solidify the therapeutic alliance, while in other clinical situations, this may not be possible or necessary.

The Dutch clinic at VU Medical Center in Amsterdam, where most empirical evidence on gender reassignment in youth is generated, uses multiple sessions stretched out over a period of time to accurately capture youth who meet criteria for GD [10]. In the United States, some providers have expressed concern that a mental health assessment protocol prior to initiating treatment may unnecessarily delay prompt treatment for the youth and that the youth will not trust the mental health provider if they feel the CAP or MHP is in a position to determine whether or not a youth should or should not receive hormone treatment [11]. Certainly this can be a valid concern, particularly when MHPs have little to no experience in working with gender diverse youth; however, a focus on training MHPs on these issues may ultimately address this gap. Therefore, it is important to recognize the barriers to care that an assessment may impose (e.g., therapeutic alliance development under the premise the provider is determining the need for gender-affirming interventions, unnecessary delay of treatment when indicated, patient access to MHPs and CAPs limitations) and mitigate those barriers through developing an assessment model that works collaboratively with the patient, family, and other providers to appropriately meet the needs of all youth presenting with gender issues.

Initially, it is important to determine the amount of sessions and time frame that those sessions take place, within the parameters of the institution or practice setting that one is treating youth in. Once that is established, then it will inform the degree to which the assessment can or cannot be comprehensive. For example, a 60-min one-session evaluation likely does not give the provider enough time to meet with the family all together, meet with the parents and child separately, obtain a diagnosis (or a list of diagnoses), come up with a gender-informed biopsychosocial formulation, and determine the appropriateness of interventions. On the other hand, for some youth who present with multiple complex issues, it can take many months in order to gain diagnostic clarity. Therefore, the task is to determine the number of sessions, length of time over which those sessions take place, and recognize what is and is not possible to determine from that structure.

For example, one structure that is used by one of the authors (Leibowitz) sets up two initial visits separated by 1 week apart: a 90-min initial visit and a subsequent 608 (THIS SHOULD SAY 60, not 608)-min visit. The 90-min initial visit is within the parameters of the amount of time allotted for an initial assessment visit by the institution. Then, typically a third visit is scheduled 4 to 6 weeks later. At some point in the initial two visits, meeting together with the family and alone separately with the parents and youth would be important. Since understanding whether or not there is the presence of gender dysphoria involves discussing sensitive information like sex anatomy and a detailed sexuality history, reserving these aspects of the interview for the second visit has proven to be more useful once the adolescent has a sense of who the provider is and some initial trust has been established. However, waiting too long in between the first and second visit may then make it more difficult in the second visit to ask about these sensitive topics considering a significant amount of time has lapsed. Another structure used by one of the other authors (Janssen) sets up an initial 3-h visit split into sections for the youth alone, the parents alone, and the family all together which is preceded by use of standardized screening, intake, and psychodiagnostic forms. The elements of the intervention and the ability to build a relationship with a patient and family over time are more important than the structure itself; however, we as clinicians must all be flexible enough to understand when a particular structure is not working and to adapt to best meet the needs of the youth and their family.

Developmental Considerations

The approach to a gender-informed biopsychosocial assessment of children and adolescents both should consider the same outcomes: promoting positive emotional, psychological, and social functioning. However, developmental differences should take into account that recommended treatment interventions differ depending on whether the youth is prepubertal, pubertal, or postpubertal.

For prepubertal children, since medical interventions are not recommended treatment interventions, some of the main focuses include (1) gender development constructs from an early age (play, clothing, toys, peer preferences, verbalization of a different gender); (2) parental beliefs and attitudes toward gender diversity; (3) other potential co-occurring psychiatric diagnoses; (4) child's understanding of the meaning of gender (and potential sources for how the child internalized the meaning of gender); (5) degree of social gender transition (change in use of pronouns, name, living in a different gender role), if pursued; (6) parent-child interactions and family dynamics; (7) psychosocial factors (school, peers, community, friends); (8) strengths and resiliency (areas where the child succeeds); and (9) individual challenges (maladaptive coping styles, rigidity, externalizing behaviors). Much of the time with the family would be with the parents alone to obtain a detailed history. However, an age-appropriate assessment with the child should attempt to elicit these constructs through typical age-appropriate assessment modalities that are used in a psychiatric assessment of a child presenting with any other issue.

For pubertal children and adolescents, the timing of the assessment is most crucial considering the intervention that would be considered for these youth meeting criteria for GD – pubertal suppression – is time dependent in terms of optimizing its effect. As described in Chap. 3 in this book ("Transgender Adolescents and the Gender Affirming Interventions: Pubertal Suppression, Hormones, Surgery, and Other Pharmacological Interventions"), if timed correctly, pubertal suppression can reversibly pause the irreversible development of secondary sex characteristics for adolescents with gender dysphoria. This may prevent unwanted anatomical changes and thus eliminate the need for more invasive procedures later on in life, should the adolescent ultimately pursue additional gender reassignment interventions as they mature psychologically and cognitively. One challenge with this age group is that pubertal onset can vary widely in terms of age. Some children who are as young as age 8 or 9 can begin puberty yet would not be emotionally or cognitively mature enough to participate in a complex interview about gender identity and sexuality issues as a 12- or 13-year-old adolescent would. Therefore, with physical and psychological maturity not necessarily in sync, it is important to be able to tailor the assessment in a way that can elicit the necessary information in order to develop a gender-informed treatment plan. This may resemble an interview that would be done for a child, or it may resemble an interview that is done with a younger adolescent, depending on the psychological maturity of the patient at hand.

An adolescent in the midst of or beyond puberty could be presenting seeking hormonal or surgical interventions. Depending on whether or not there are co-occurring psychiatric conditions (e.g., an adolescent with autism spectrum disorder might be more concrete and therefore understand gender identity-related constructs on more concrete levels), the approach to an adolescent with gender identity concerns should not differ much from the approach to any other adolescent. What differs is whether or not the adolescent is seeking irreversible treatments, meets criteria for gender dysphoria, and/or has family support for such interventions when they are indeed clinically appropriate.

Collateral Information

The Endocrine Society Guidelines [4] emphasize the importance of multidisciplinary collaboration when possible. The psychiatrist, both trained in medical and psychological aspects of health, can often serve as a conduit between MHPs and medical providers for youth with gender dysphoria.

In the assessment phase of treatment, important information from a pediatrician would be the degree of pubertal maturation that has taken place for a given child or adolescent. For youth who have existing therapists, two tasks are important for the CAP: (1) determining the extent to which gender identity-related issues have been explored in therapy and if so (2) what has taken place in therapy thus far regarding diagnostic clarity, family dynamics, and any other co-occurring conditions that the child or adolescent may have. Some MHPs may have referred the patient to the CAP with a specific intention (e.g., as noted above, to assess "readiness" for a gender-affirming treatment or perhaps for a psychopharmacological intervention). It is important to obtain an entire picture of the youth and family that includes the typical biopsychosocial factors obtained in a routine psychiatric assessment *in addition to* aspects related to the gender. The biopsychosocial factors provide a context for the psychiatrist that will assist in procuring diagnostic clarity and developing an appropriate initial treatment plan.

Documentation

Standard documentation does not include ways to address gender-related concerns in a psychiatric assessment. In order to document properly, using the most appropriate pronoun set and name, it is important to consider the clinical situation and the fact that the parent(s) or guardian(s) are ultimately able to receive the psychiatric assessment should they request it. Therefore, aspects of the assessment that are shared privately by the adolescent may need to be summarized in a way that prioritizes safety for the youth should the clinician believe that parental access to the record could lead to an unsafe situation.

Interviewing About Gender Identity

The initial interview should ask open-ended questions about gender identity, expression, and sexual orientation. Developmental considerations should be taken into account, appropriate to how a child or adolescent is able to conceptualize these different aspects of their sense of self. We want to understand how an individual understands their identity, their body, how gender impacts their role in society and in their relationships, and how they may wish for these things to remain the same or change. Questions that do not make presumptions about how a particular child or adolescent thinks about these issues are more likely to yield valuable clinical information.

Table 1.4 Possible interview questions for the prepubertal child

Establishing meaning of gender to the child
• Tell me what it means to be a boy and what it means to be a girl. • Is it possible to be something other than a boy or a girl?
Specific questions about the child
• Are *you* a boy or a girl [or whatever the child says above]? • What is it like for you when you are with boys or girls who are different types of boys or girls than you are? • Can boys like [list things the child typically associates with girls]? • Can girls like [list things child typically associates with boys]? • What types of activities and toys do *you* like to do and play with? • Do you like to have friends who are boys, girls, or both?

Questions for the Prepubertal Child

Children typically think in concrete terms. Understanding the meaning of gender for the child provides context around the answers to questions that a child would provide when asked about gender. It may be helpful to consider inserting these types of questions into a game that includes questions that ask the child about other areas of their life, including but not limited to their friends, hobbies, school, family life, favorite games, etc. By *not* making gender the exclusive focus of the interview, it may put the child at ease and allow the clinician to explore these issues without making the child uncomfortable, in particular if the issues are uncomfortable for the child in the first place. Other children may relish the opportunity to speak with an interested adult about their gender and may take little to no time to warm up to the assessment. Table 1.4 includes potential initial questions to consider when assessing gender issues in a prepubertal child.

Questions for the Adolescent

The adolescent may or may not feel comfortable discussing gender issues, depending on who is present in the room. Therefore, as is typical in the psychiatric interview with all adolescents, assessing gender-related concepts requires spending time with the adolescent alone. Table 1.5 includes potential questions to consider when assessing gender issues in an adolescent.

Clarifying these questions may give the clinician an opportunity to explore *why* an adolescent feels the way they do. The last set of questions help explore the adolescent's perception of the advantages and disadvantages experienced by the different genders within a particular society. This helps the provider delineate whether the adolescent can appreciate the variety aspects of being a particular gender for all the genders, not just the gender they were assigned at birth or the gender they identify as. The answers may also give the provider a sense as to how sophisticated the adolescent's thinking is about different gender roles and how societal definitions of gender

Table 1.5 Possible interview questions for the adolescent

Initial questions with the parent(s) present
Say: "I will have a chance to ask you these questions without your parent/guardian if you feel that will be helpful." • What name for yourself do you feel most comfortable using? • What pronoun do you feel most comfortable with me using to refer to you? • Are there situations where this might change?
Initial questions without the parent(s) present
Say: "Now that we are alone I am going to ask you some more questions." • What name for yourself do you feel most comfortable using in private? • What pronoun do you feel most comfortable with me using to refer to you? • Would this change depending on who you are with? • Is there a gender you feel most comfortable identifying as? • Are there aspects of the gender you were assigned to at birth that you feel comfortable with? Uncomfortable with? • Are there aspects of another gender that you feel comfortable with? Uncomfortable with? • Are there aspects of maleness that you relate to? What about femaleness?
More personal questions for the adolescent without the parent(s) present
Say: "I am now going to ask you questions about your body and please let me know if you are comfortable answering the questions or not." • Are there any aspects of your body that you are comfortable with? Which ones? • Are there any aspects of your body that you are uncomfortable with? Which ones? • Are they any aspects of your body that you would want to change? Which ones? • Are there any aspects of the body of a different gender that you desire? Which ones? • Are there any aspects of the body of a different gender that you do not desire? Which ones?
Questions to help understand adolescent perceptions of different gender role advantages and disadvantages
• What are the advantages that females experience in society? • What are the disadvantages that females experience in society? • What are the advantages that males experience in society? • What are the disadvantages that males experience in society? • What are the advantages that nonbinary people experience in society? • What are the disadvantages that nonbinary people experience in society? • What are the advantages that people with no gender experience in society? • What are the disadvantages that people with no gender experience in society?

play a role into the adolescent's thinking about gender. One adolescent might have a very rigid idea about what the advantages and disadvantages are for a particular gender, yet another might demonstrate marked sophistication and flexibility about different genders within a particular society.

Assessment Constructs

Two review articles in a 2016 International Review of Psychiatry edition on gender dysphoria provide a detailed overview of the assessment aims across both childhood [12] and adolescence [13]. In this chapter, specific details regarding five main areas of assessment are described. These constructs are specific to gender. However, obtaining an overall clinical picture of the youth and family by doing a typical psychodiagnostic assessment is equally important as noted in the WPATH Standards of Care [5].

Pronoun and Name Use

For youth presenting with gender-related concerns, perhaps one of the most challenging yet effective approach to the work is to focus on pronouns and name use, both in the assessment and in an ongoing way. This is not based on empirical data or scientific study. However, the provider who demonstrates awareness that pronouns and names can differ from those associated with the child or adolescent's given name and gender is already very much ahead of the providers who do not.

Assessment and use of the appropriate pronoun set and name involves nuanced decision-making, depending on who is in the room. Developing therapeutic rapport with the young person presenting with a gender-related concern is more likely to be achieved faster if the provider introduces themselves with their preferred name (e.g., "My name is Dr. Leibowitz, but I also go by Dr. Scott") and pronoun set (e.g., "when people refer to me, I feel most comfortable when they use male pronouns: he him, and his."). More often than not, asking everyone in the room to introduce themselves with a chosen name and set of pronouns sets the stage for a clinical treatment frame that shows sensitivity to individuals who may identify as another gender. In other situations, when it may be identified prior (through an intake staffer or administrative staff) that a parent is highly averse to gender diversity, it might be reasonable for the provider to use clinical judgment whether or not an introduction that focuses on pronouns and potentially a different name for the adolescent should be used.

Observing affect in the room between parents and their adolescent when assessing pronouns and chosen name yields valuable clinical information regarding the dynamics of the family around this issue. In some situations the youth may use their birth name and pronouns associated with their assigned sex at birth, yet at another point in the assessment when meeting alone with them, it is important to ask again and assess whether or not their answers change and why.

As time with the family progresses, determining when to use which pronouns and name requires careful consideration so as not to isolate any one member of the family. There are a myriad of situations in which the use of pronouns and name can change, depending on the circumstances at the time. There is no empirical data regarding the best way to approach this issue, so Table 1.6 presents only a small number of the possible clinical situations that can arise and potential ways to approach it based on anecdotal experience from the authors. In some situations, the clinician may find themselves needing to avoid using pronouns and names altogether in order to maintain a positive therapeutic alliance with the parent(s) or guardian(s). In other situations, it may be worthwhile to challenge the parent or

Table 1.6 Pronoun and name use scenarios based on family dynamics

Scenario	Pronoun and name intervention
Parent(s) highly opposed and adolescent is open in front of them	• Assess affect in the room and consider splitting the parents from the adolescent • When alone with parents, ask what pronouns and name most sense for you to use when with them • Educate support staff to avoid use of pronoun and name as much as possible and/or ask the parent what name and pronouns makes most sense to be using when referring to the adolescent
Parent(s) highly opposed and adolescent is not open in front of them	• Assess affect in the room and use pronouns and name that everyone is in agreement with when all together • Privately with the adolescent, ask what pronouns and name to use with them, with parents alone, and with them all together • Assess why adolescent feels uncomfortable being open in front of parents • Educate support staff to avoid use of pronoun and name as much as possible and/or ask the parent what name and pronouns makes most sense to be using when referring to the adolescent
Parent(s) supportive and adolescent is open in front of them	• Use pronouns and name that everyone is using • Educate support staff to use agreed upon pronouns and name when referring to adolescent
Parent(s) supportive and adolescent is not open in front of them	• Use pronouns and name that everyone is using • When privately with adolescent, assess why they are not open with their supportive parents when all together • Educate support staff to use pronouns and name that adolescent desires
Parent(s) aware and supportive of gender identity issue for a long time and not using pronoun or correct name	• Assess how parents use of birth-assigned name and associated pronouns affect adolescent • When alone with parents, assess what the barriers are to using adolescent's chosen name and/or pronouns • Educate support staff to use pronouns and name that adolescent desires
Parent(s) using desired pronouns and name in some situation but not in others	• When alone with parents, assess intentions of parents • Assess why there is discrepant use of chosen name and pronouns in different situations • Educate support staff to use pronouns and/or name that adolescent desires
Parent(s) refusing to use desired pronouns and this has introduced an element of control between parent(s) and adolescent	• Consider educating parents about the potential negative effects of the lack of using the adolescent's desired pronouns and/or name • Consider framing parental attempts to use adolescent desired pronouns and/or name as a means of *exploring* how the adolescent responds to being perceived in the way the adolescent desires

guardian to use the correct or chosen pronoun and/or name, considering a fair amount of time has gone by since the youth has begun using this name and it is clear that gender transition is going to promote positive emotional, psychological, and social functioning.

Gender Identity, Gender Expression, and Sexual Orientation

One key aspect in the assessment of these youth is to understand the child or adolescent's developmentally appropriate understanding of the difference between gender identity, gender expression, and sexual orientation. For adolescents, sexual arousal, fantasies, and experimentation behaviors may begin to emerge. Many transgender youth will not engage in sexual activity or behavior because they are uncomfortable with these aspects of their body. On the other hand, understanding how the youth sees themselves as a sexual being could potentially help them recognize aspects about their gender that they might not have thought about. For example, if a youth has a strict notion about certain gender roles being associated with specific sexual behaviors (e.g., whether the message that they have received in their upbringing has been that a man *must be* with a woman or that a man has to be in a sexually dominant role), it is important to rule out the possibility that these notions are influencing the youth's self-concept of their gender identity.

Depending on a variety of factors, whether it be cognitive, developmental, or reactions to environmental messages about gender, it is possible that these phenomena can be conflated by the youth and/or their family members. The following vignettes illustrate this possibility:

> A 7-year-old assigned male at birth presents in clinical practice affirming a female gender identity. The child's parents are using male pronouns to refer to him and want to know whether or not their child is transgender. They state "he likes wearing dresses, playing with dolls, and only wants to be princess characters when playing with his peers." The provider spends time playing with the child and intersperses questions about gender into a game. During the game, the child psychiatrist puts a boy figure into a dress and the child says, "Boys cannot wear dresses, silly! That's only for girls."

This is an example of a prepubertal child who has internalized binary gender roles that are associated with one particular gender. The provider can use this opportunity to ask "*Is it possible for boys to wear dresses?*" with an aim to understand a child's cognitive flexibility and begin to tease apart the differences between identity and role. Notably, both cisgender and transgender youth alike will often internalize binary gender roles, and helping children to explore their ideas around gender roles can help clarify the underlying gender identity.

> A parent of a 16-year-old transgender female seeking estrogen treatment asks to speak with the clinician privately. The parent, who has been making strides in accepting her new daughter (previously a son) appears distressed. She tells the clinician "I just caught him, I mean her, with pictures on her phone kissing another girl. If she is interested in girls, then I don't understand why she cannot simply just go back to be a boy? Maybe she's just a boy and not transgender after all. Help!"

In this situation, the parent is not recognizing that all individuals – both cisgender and transgender alike – can have same-gender attractions and engage in same-gender sexual behaviors. Validating the parent's confusion may be a starting point.

It may help the parent feel the MHP understand their dilemma. As the parent develops trust with the MHP, further education about the difference between gender identity and sexual orientation may be understood and appreciated better.

A 14-year-old depressed assigned female at birth with autism spectrum disorder presents in clinical practice seeking testosterone therapy. The patient has been binding his chest and is using male pronouns. You ask him how he felt about being perceived as female and he responds with, "Every time I would wear a dress or makeup, people would stare at me and it would make me uncomfortable. Guys don't have to deal with that. I think being a guy is easier."

In this situation, the adolescent may be approaching their thinking about gender in concrete ways that are not typical for an adolescent. They may also be having difficulty communicating their inner experiences accurately. Often adolescents with autism spectrum disorder (although not limited to that population) can think in concrete ways, and so ensuring that they are not conflating the concept of *being another gender* from *ideas about how particular genders are expressed* is important to distinguish.

A 12-year-old assigned male at birth presents in clinical practice living in a rural area where homosexuality is widely considered a "negative lifestyle." He presents as very effeminate and enjoys experimenting with makeup, which has elicited punishment from his parents who believe that this type of behavior is a sin. He opens up to his provider revealing that he has attractions to other boys and does not feel anything for girls other than wanting to be friends with them. He says, "I think this means I might be a girl since it just is not allowed for boys to like boys in that way."

In this situation, the young adolescent may be conflating sexual orientation with gender identity and gender expression. He may also not be. However, it is important for the provider to be able to understand what is at the root of his assertion. Has it been ingrained in his mind that being gay is a significantly negative thing that will lead him to have a bad life? Is he thinking that because he has these attractions that it *must mean* he is a girl or should be a girl? Is he aware that individuals who are born male could potentially be female, something different than having attractions to males as male?

A parent of a 14-year-old assigned female at birth who presents stating "I am a boy," asks to speak with the provider quietly. The parent states, "she's always been more masculine and I don't understand this whole transgender thing. To me, she's just a lesbian."

In this scenario, the parent appears to be connecting the adolescent's more masculine appearance and mannerisms with a particular sexual orientation. The vignette does not describe the assessment of the adolescent in detail, so on its own, this example simply demonstrates a parent who is making a false association between gender expression and sexual orientation. If the adolescent in fact meets criteria for gender dysphoria and identifies consistently as male, then working through the parent's understanding of the different phenomena would be a target intervention.

Family Dynamics

More globally, family systems theory recognizes the influence that individual transitions within family systems can affect the entire family [14, 15]. This is no different for transgender youth, and it has been demonstrated that caregivers significantly affect emotional well-being for them [16]. In the Trans Youth Family Study, data that comes from a series of qualitative interviews of children, adolescents, and family members, Katz-Wise et al. describe seven overarching themes that are crucial to transgender youths' identity development. One of these themes is family adjustment/impact [17]. The study illustrates that the range in which caregivers express their reactions and emotions to the child or adolescent impacts the way in which they provide support and ultimately how that affects the youth's own ability to navigate being gender diverse in society today.

For youth who exist as gender nonconforming (without transitioning to another gender, per se), youth who seek to transition to another gender (but who do not for any number of reasons), and/or youth who are in the process of transitioning to a different gender, the implications that these situations might have on the family dynamic as a whole are important to consider. Describing the various permutations that exist with factors that include family constellations, reactions of different family members, emotions of different family members, and effects that gender diversity might have on a given family system is clearly not possible. However, it is important for the psychiatrist or mental health provider to have a sense as to where each person in the family might be in terms of their belief systems, emotions, and reactions to gender diversity and gender transition in order to help ensure psychological and physical safety for the youth.

Clinically, assessment of the family dynamic is therefore important. Depending on the family, some communication patterns between family members might be obvious after only one or two sessions, while in others it may take more time to understand. Chapter 4 (MacNish) in this book demonstrates a case where family dynamics poses a challenge and the way the situation was approached. Table 1.7 lists some situations that may arise and the treatment aims that might accompany the scenario.

Coping Strategies

All youth present with differing ways to manage stress. Some are resilient, others less so, and most youth utilize a mixture of both healthy and unhealthy coping strategies in the face of adversity and stigma. One youth might shut down and become nonverbal. Another might begin to engage in risk-taking behaviors. Other youth may come to the realization that waiting until they are older in order to transition genders makes most sense for them. Whether the adolescent becomes depressed, anxious, or starts to act out and become oppositional, it is important for the clinician to factor in the relationship between these coping strategies and gender identity.

Table 1.7 Possible scenarios involving differing family dynamics

Caregiver reactions	Diagnostic formulation	Potential treatment aim beyond assessment
Both parents supportive of medical transition	Gender dysphoria of adolescence (definitive)	• Work through family expectations of the changes that will happen • Work through how parents can support the youth and each other
One parent is supportive and one parent is adamantly against medical gender transition	Gender dysphoria of adolescence (definitive)	• Consider working through parent disagreement and conflict that may arise between them • Consider working with the parent who is against transition to shift from completely against to partially against or even neutral
Both parents are fearful of gender transition	Gender dysphoria of adolescence (definitive)	• Consider exploration with parents about their fears, both separately and together • Consider the effect that the parental fear has on the adolescent's emotional well-being
One parent is supportive and the other is skeptical, thinking this is "a phase"	Gender dysphoria of adolescence (definitive)	• Consider working with the skeptical parent to gain a better understanding of the skepticism • Consider intervening if it is determined that the gender issue • Consider the effect that the differing views have on the adolescent
Parents are aligned that the adolescent's declared gender identity is "a phase"	Gender dysphoria of childhood or adolescence (provisional)	• Consider a therapy plan that helps establish more clarity on the diagnosis of the child or adolescent (identifying reasons why it may not be definitive) • Consider working with parents to understand if their skepticism itself is playing a role in the diagnostic uncertainty (e.g., reaction of adolescent to parents who do not accept them)
Parent(s) believe(s) the youth is transgender	Gender exploring child or adolescent	• Consider working with the parent to help allow the child or adolescent explore their gender identity and expression without any one trajectory • Consider working with the parent to understand more about their interpretation of the child or adolescent's behavior
Parent(s) do(es) not believe the youth is transgender	Gender dysphoria of childhood or adolescence (definitive)	• Consider further assessment of parent(s) belief system and why they may feel differently from the clinician • Consider additional modalities to help provide psychoeducation to parent while maintaining a therapeutic alliance

Healthy and unhealthy coping strategies could influence the way others perceive the adolescent and the gender that the youth asserts. Therefore, recognizing whether the coping strategy is a barrier to being perceived authentically is a task of the provider. For example, a youth with gender dysphoria who avoids confrontation and is frequently referred to as the birth name yet refuses to correct the person could reinforce a belief in the other person that the youth "must not be transgender since if it were the case, wouldn't they be correcting me every time I used the wrong name?" On the other hand, a youth who tends to consistently react excessively and disproportionately in response to mild stressors, a pronoun or name correction could be misinterpreted by others as "that's just Jimmy being Jimmy again. He responds to EVERYTHING in such a dramatic way." Therefore, the provider must take into account the temperament, coping strategies, and ways that the youth are resilient when addressing the way others perceive them.

Similarly, the coping strategies of the adolescent could also influence the way in which they manage a gender transition, should that be appropriate. For youth who begin treatment with hormones, subtle changes to their body will occur over time. While these changes may be desired by the adolescent, there are a variety of possible reactions that may develop, both within the adolescent as well as for others in the adolescent's life. For example, the youth who tends to react impulsively in response to perceived slights might not be prepared to navigate others' responses to their changing body. Another youth who is avoidant of difficult conversations may not appreciate the importance of disclosure to close family members (perhaps with the help of supportive parents) that he has started testosterone and therefore cannot anticipate how to navigate a situation where an unknowing family reacts to him with surprise once his voice starts to lower or facial hair begins to develop.

Therefore, for all youth with gender-related concerns, understanding the way they cope interpersonally is both useful when assisting both being perceived in an authentic way but also navigating potential changes that can arise for those moving forward with medical and/or surgical gender transition.

Psychosocial and Community Factors

The youth's community, school, and extended family members are all important components to assess with respect to gender-related concerns. Certain school climates are supportive of youth who are gender diverse and/or transgender. They allow for these youth to use facilities that are consistent with the gender that the youth affirms. Such schools may change the youth's name in a roster, have an extracurricular group that provides the youth the opportunity to meet other students who are going through similar issues, and/or have teachers refer to the youth by the pronoun and name that is most correct for them. On the other hand, other schools may take a rigid stance about the way they approach gender, often equating an individual's sex with their gender. Understanding the school climate provides important information to the MHP or CAP.

Additionally, evaluating the degree of support or rejection that the community and extended family members provide to the youth can provide important details necessary to formulate a treatment plan. Often, caregivers may be afraid of the reactions of their extended family members if their child is gender nonconforming and/or transgender, and then this might shape how they interact with the youth. On the other hand, the youth may not want extended family members to know about their gender identity or desire to transition, and this can create complex situations for the immediate family. For example, an adolescent may expect their parents to use one set of pronouns within the confines of their home, yet when they are among community or extended family members, the youth may want the parents to revert back to a different pronoun set. This has the potential to be confusing to parents and families. Therefore, understanding the nuance of the various external factors that could influence the youth's emotional and psychological functioning requires assessment of those various aspects of life for the child.

Psychometric Instruments

Standardized instruments have been developed and used to assist in diagnostic assessment for youth presenting with gender identity concerns. A more comprehensive review of these measures can be found in Zucker [18]. With the shift in the DSM approaching gender identity as a spectrum (from dichotomous categories), as well as youth presenting having already partially or fully transitioned to a different gender, many of the validated instruments across development are not as clinically useful as they once may have been. Some of the questions that ask about what it is like to live in the gender role of their assigned gender at birth presume that an individual has not transitioned and, therefore, an adolescent who has already partially or fully socially transitioned could rate a lower level of distress in response to such questions. Additionally, as adolescents transition through use of evidence-based gender-affirming treatments, anatomical features may change, and therefore some of the instruments may not be able to be administered over time (e.g., a female version of a body inventory might not include facial hair as an anatomical component, and so with the development of facial hair that comes with testosterone, the instrument would not capture the adolescent's level of satisfaction with that secondary sex characteristic). Therefore, it is highly recommended to consult with a psychologist, psychiatrist, or other MHP who is knowledgeable about the utility of the gender-specific instruments before using them to guide an assessment. Developing new measures that appreciate the complexity of the current landscape of clinical practice is an area of current research.

Psychometric Instruments for Children

For prepubertal children, there is an interview known as the Gender Identity Interview for Children [19] and a questionnaire about Gender Identity Questionnaire for Children [20]. The GIIC is a 12-item child informant instrument that measures two factors: "cognitive gender confusion" and "affective gender confusion" [19]. Cognitive gender confusion is assessed by four questions asking whether the child identifies as a boy or a girl (e.g., "When you grow up, will you be a mommy or a daddy?"). Affective gender confusion is assessed by eight questions such as "Are there things that you don't like about being a boy?" Additionally, projective tests such as the Draw-a-Person test [21] has been used to help in aiding whether the child sees themselves as female or male.

Psychometric Instruments for Adolescents

With adolescents, there are a handful of validated instruments that have been used to aid in the assessment of youth presenting with gender-related concerns. They include, but are not limited to, the following: (1) Utrecht Gender Dysphoria Scale (UGDS), which is a twelve-question, five-point Likert scale (range 12–60) with two versions, one for assigned males and one for assigned females at birth [22]; (2) Body Image Scale, which is a dimensional assessment of body dysphoria by asking the adolescent to assess satisfaction with different anatomical features of their body in addition to whether or not they would want to change that feature [23]; and (3) the Gender Minority Stress and Resilience Scale (GMSR), which assesses for nine constructs related to minority stress, resilience, acceptance, and expectations of the future as a gender minority individual [24].

Assessing for Appropriateness for Hormonal and/or Surgical Interventions

The WPATH Standards of Care 7th edition provides criteria for hormonal and surgical interventions [5], which are listed in Table 1.8. The interventions are discussed in more detail in Chap. 3. These interventions are only applicable to adolescents or psychologically mature individuals who are at Tanner stage 2 of puberty or beyond.

As noted above, when the frame of the assessment is exclusively about determining the appropriateness of medical and/or surgical interventions to address gender dysphoria, it is important to take into account the power imbalance that exists between the adolescent and provider. For an adolescent seeking a hormonal or surgical intervention, meeting with the provider under this specific premise can viewed as a *means to an end*, which itself can impact what is and is not disclosed.

Table 1.8 Criteria for interventions according to World Professional Association of Transgender Health, Standards of Care 7th edition; with stipulations from 2017 Endocrine Society Guidelines

Intervention	Criteria with minors
Most reversible Pubertal suppression with gonadotropin-releasing hormone agonists	• Persistent and pervasive history of gender nonconformity or gender dysphoria • Gender dysphoria emerged or worsened with the onset of puberty • Co-occurring psychological, medical, or social difficulties that might interfere with treatment are addressed • Adolescent and family have given informed consent
Partially reversible Masculinizing or feminizing hormones (testosterone and estrogen)	• Persistent, well-documented gender dysphoria • Capacity to make a fully informed decision to consent for treatment • Age of majority (which is 16 in many countries), however with parental consent, this can be younger. Per Endocrine Society Guidelines, the age could be lower depending on the maturity and sophistication of the adolescent • If significant medical or mental health concerns are present, they must be reasonably well controlled
Irreversible Surgical	*Criteria for surgery* • Persistent well-documented gender dysphoria • Capacity to make a fully informed decision and to consent for treatment • Age of majority (which is 16 years old in many countries), however in the United States, 16 years old with parental consent is typical for chest surgery • If significant medical or mental health concerns are present, they must be reasonably well controlled *Chest surgery* • One referral letter is necessary from a mental health professional • Preferably after ample time living in desired gender role • Preferably after 1 year of testosterone treatment (however there is flexibility built into the standards of care depending on an adolescent's specific clinical situation and goals for gender identity expression) *Genital surgery* • Two referral letters from mental health providers are necessary • Recommend that patients reach legal age of majority in a given country • Recommend that patients have lived continuously for at least 12 months in the gender role that is congruent with their gender identity • Recommend being on hormone therapy for at least 1 year prior to the surgery

Often, youth may believe that their provider will prevent access from treatments that they believe are important for their emotional and physical health. This may lead to a minimization of disclosure of psychiatric symptoms. It can also lead to youth falsely describing a binary gender identity when in fact they may experience aspects of both male and female identities. Therefore, establishing trust with the adolescent and family is of paramount importance. As noted above, it may be important to reframe the assessment aim as a collaborative process that prioritizes the shared goal of an emotionally, psychologically, and socially healthy adolescent which *may or may not* involve medical interventions.

As the provider considers the benefit of these medical and/or surgical interventions, the individual clinical situation should be factored into account. Determining the presence of GD can be difficult to ascertain without a complete biopsychosocial understanding of the adolescent. There are certain situations that may cloud the ability to understand whether or not the adolescent meets criteria for GD, which can include (1) co-occurring psychiatric diagnoses, (2) family conflict that may influence an adolescent's assertion, (3) temperament and psychological factors of the adolescent, and (4) cognitive aspects of the adolescent that may lead them to conflate phenomena described above (gender identity, gender expression, and/or sexual orientation). In these situations when a medical or surgical intervention is sought by an adolescent, addressing these issues in treatment would help distinguish whether or not the adolescent meets criteria definitively for GD. Until then, it would be important to consider the adolescent as meeting the criteria *provisionally* if they endorse the criteria as noted above. There are reversible interventions described in Chap. 3, such as an androgen-blocking agent (spironolactone for the transfeminine population) or a menstrual suppression agent (progestin for the transmasculine population) that can help alleviate some aspects of undesired physical symptoms, which may help buy time to further clarify whether criteria are in fact met, yet also affirm the adolescent in addressing their needs.

For adolescents who definitively meet the criteria for GD and seek these interventions, the issue then becomes *appropriate timing* of the intervention. Withholding an intervention is not a neutral act, so therefore it is important to ensure that adolescents are referred to the appropriate medical specialist within a reasonable time frame. One key aspect that has become increasingly important to explore in treatment before the provision of medical interventions would be fertility. Most transgender adolescents seeking hormonal intervention are not interested in pursuing fertility preservation [25], especially since there is a lack of insurance coverage for what can be a costly endeavor. However, understanding all family members' perceptions on fertility and managing those expectations would be important to navigate prior to the use of interventions that affect fertility.

Therefore, issues that might impair readiness for these interventions even in a situation where GD criteria are definitively met may include (1) acute unstable psychiatric concerns (e.g., but not limited to active suicidality, active self-injury, psychotic processes, mania, and/or profound anxiety that acutely impairs the functioning of the adolescent); (2) challenging family dynamics where parents are unwilling to consent for one reason or another; (3) fertility desires have not been addressed; (4) inability to understand the benefits, risks, effects, and timeline of effects of the interventions; (5) false expectations about the effects of the interventions; and (6) a significant predictable psychosocial stressor that may make initiation of the intervention more stressful than beneficial. Helping the youth and families think through the consequences of the various interventions requires the CAP or MHP to understand the effects and management needs of the interventions. For example, a youth starting testosterone will need to have lab work done and need to be able to understand the delivery methods for the hormone (e.g., can be challenging for a youth with a needle phobia). For older adolescents moving forward with chest surgery, not understanding the aftercare needs (e.g., the need for rest with the presence of chest drains and wound management) can interfere with postoperative course.

Therefore, in order to provide timely treatment for these sought after interventions where timing or readiness factors may delay the initiation of the intervention, it is important to collaboratively prioritize those factors as treatment goals. In this sense, the MHP or CAP can serve as a *collaborative path paver* instead of viewed upon as the sole decision-maker, which often leads the adolescent to perceive the provider as someone standing in the way of accessing important treatments that will reduce their suffering.

Consultation with the endocrinologist or pediatric gender specialist provider would potentially be a useful tool to help the youth and family receive answers to questions about the interventions they are seeking. A discussion with the provider *prior to* the appointment may be useful to help coordinate the care and provide the medical provider an understanding of the biopsychosocial factors that may influence the timing of the interventions so that false expectations and mixed messages are not delivered to the adolescent and family. An initial psychoeducation visit on the side effects, risks, benefits, and timeline of effects of the interventions may be very useful for the adolescent and family. It is noted that counseling patients to consider the potential iatrogenic harms of hormone therapy is an important ethical consideration [26]. A subsequent visit with the mental health provider, whether it be as part of the initial assessment phase or later on during the treatment phase, could then determine whether or not the adolescent and/or family was able to absorb the information provided to them by the medical provider sufficient enough to provide informed assent and consent.

Conclusion

The approach to the assessment for children and adolescents presenting with gender identity-related concerns is complex. It requires the CAP or MHP to be aware of numerous factors that are both specific to gender and those that are related to the typical psychodiagnostic assessment done for all youth. Not only should the assessment capture aspects within each of these two broad categories, but understanding the interplay between the general functioning of the youth and the gender identity issues that they present with adds another layer of complexity. To leave it at that would still oversimply the assessment as the provider must also consider developmental aspects of gender, the desired medical and surgical interventions that the adolescent may want, and the complex nuanced aspect of interpersonal communication (through pronouns and name) that is often taken for granted when gender issues are not a part of a treatment frame. This initial chapter lays the groundwork for the provider to approach an assessment that is affirmative, gender-informed, developmentally informed, and guides the development of a treatment plan that prioritizes timely access to evidence-based gender-affirming interventions in the population of youth for whom they are clinically indicated and appropriate.

References

1. American Psychiatric Association. Diagnostic and statistical manual of mental disorders. 5th ed. Arlington, VA: American Psychiatric Association; 2013.
2. Hsieh S, Leininger J. Resource list: clinical care programs for gender-nonconforming children and adolescents. Pediatric Ann. 2014;43(6):238–44. https://doi.org/10.3928/00904481-20140522-11.
3. Adelson SL. American Academy of Child and Adolescent Psychiatry (AACAP) Committee on Quality Issues (CQI). Practice parameter on gay, lesbian or bisexual sexual orientation, gender-nonconformity, and gender discordance in children and adolescents. J Am Acad Child Adolesc Psychiatry. 2012;51(9):957–74.
4. Hembree WC, Cohen-Kettenis PT, Gooren L, Hannema SE, Meyer WJ, Murad MH, et al. Endocrine treatment of gender-dysphoric/gender-incongruent persons: an Endocrine Society* clinical practice guideline. J Clin Endocrinol Metab. 2017;102(11):3869–903. https://doi.org/10.1210/jc.2017-01658.
5. Coleman E, Bockting W, Botzer M, Cohen-Kettenis P, DeCuypere G, Feldman J, et al. Standards of care for the health of transsexual, transgender, and gender-nonconforming people, version 7. Int J Transgenderism. 2012;13(4):165–232.
6. Wallien MS, Swaab H, Cohen-Kettenis PT. Psychiatric comorbidity among children with gender identity disorder. J Am Acad Child Adolesc Psychiatry. 2007;46(10):1307–14.
7. Meyer IH. Prejudice, social stress, and mental health in lesbian, gay, and bisexual populations: conceptual issues and research evidence. Psychol Bull. 2003;129(5):674–97.
8. Hendricks ML, Testa RJ. A conceptual framework for clinical work with transgender and gender nonconforming clients: an adaptation of the minority stress model. Prof Psychol Res Pr. 2012;43(5):460–7.
9. Grant J, Mottet L, Tanis J, Harrison J, Herman J, Keisling M. Injustice at every turn: a report of the National Transgender Discrimination Survey. Washington, DC: National Center for Transgender Equality and National Gay and Lesbian Task Force; 2011.
10. de Vries AL, Cohen-Kettenis PT. Clinical management of gender dysphoria in children and adolescents: the Dutch approach. J Homosex. 2012;59(3):301–20. https://doi.org/10.1080/00918369.2012.653300.
11. Olson-Kennedy J. Mental health disparities among transgender youth. Rethinking the role of professionals. JAMA Pediatr. 2016;170(5):423–4.
12. Ristori J, Steensma T. Gender dysphoria in childhood. Int Rev Psychiatry. 2016;28(1):13–20.
13. Leibowitz SF, de Vries ALC. Gender dysphoria in adolescence. Int Rev Psychiatry. 2016; 28(1):21–35.
14. Cox MJ, Paley B. Families as systems. Ann Rev Psychol. 1997;48:243–67. https://doi.org/10.1146/annurev.psych.48.1.243.
15. Minuchin P. Families and individual development: provocations from the field of family therapy. Child Dev. 1985;56:289–302.
16. McConnell EA, Birkett M, Mustanski B. Families matter: social support and mental health trajectories among lesbian, gay, bisexual, and transgender youth. J Adolesc Health. 2016;59: 674–80. https://doi.org/10.1016/j.jadohealth.2016.07.026.
17. Katz-Wise S, Budge S, Fugate E, Flanagan K, Touloumtzis C, Rood B, et al. Transactional pathways of transgender identity development in transgender and gender-nonconforming youth and caregiver perspectives from the trans youth family study. Int J Transgenderism. 2017;18(3):243–63. https://doi.org/10.1080/15532739.2017.1304312.

18. Zucker KJ. Measurement of psychosexual differentiation. Arch Sex Behav. 2005;34:375–88.
19. Zucker KJ, Bradley SJ, Sullivan CB, Kuksis M, Birkenfeld-Adams A, Mitchell JN. A gender identity interview for children. J Pers Assess. 1993;61:443–56.
20. Johnson LL, Bradley SJ, Birkenfeld-Adams AS, Kuksis MA, Maing DM, Mitchell JN, et al. A parent-report gender identity questionnaire for children. Arch Sex Behav. 2004;33:105–16.
21. Zucker KJ, Finegan JK, Doering RW, Bradley SJ. Human figure drawings of gender-problem children: a comparison to sibling, psychiatric, and normal controls. J Abnorm Child Psychol. 1983;11:287–98.
22. Schneider C, Cerwenska S, Nieder T, Briken P, Cohen-Kettenis PT, DeCuypere G, et al. Measuring gender dysphoria: a multicenter examination and comparison of the Utrecht gender dysphoria scale and the gender identity/gender dysphoria questionnaire for adolescents and adults. Arch Sex Behav. 2016;45(3):551–8.
23. Lindgren TW, Pauly IB. A body image scale for evaluating transsexuals. Arch Sex Behav. 1975;4(6):639–56.
24. Testa RJ, Habarth J, Peta J, Balsam K, Bockting W. Development of the gender minority stress and resilience measure. Psychol Sex Orientat Gender Diversity. 2015;2(1):65–77.
25. Nahata L, Tishelman A, Caltabellotta N, Quinn G. Low fertility preservation utilization among transgender youth. J Adolesc Health. 2017;61(1):40–4.
26. Steensma T, Wensing-Kruger S, Klink D. How should physicians help gender-transitioning adolescents consider the iatrogenic harms of hormone therapy? AMA J Ethics. 2017;19(8):762–70.

Chapter 2
Social Gender Transition and the Psychological Interventions

Scott Leibowitz

Introduction

Youth presenting with gender-related concerns and their families are increasingly presenting to mental health professionals seeking guidance. Many of these children and adolescents are presenting having already undergone a social gender transition (defined by living socially as a different gender from one's assigned gender at birth by use of different pronoun, name, clothing, etc.), either partially or fully, while some are seeking help from the mental health professional regarding how to move forward with next steps. The assessment chapter preceding this one offers details on how the mental health professional, or more specifically the child and adolescent psychiatrist, can assess for the presence of gender dysphoria. However, there may be children and adolescents without gender dysphoria who are gender diverse in their authentic expression of self as a particular gender. This chapter will provide an overview of social gender transition, other nonmedical interventions with psychological effects, and the different considerations that a provider might factor in across developmental stages, when providing gender-affirming care to children, adolescents, and their families.

S. Leibowitz, MD
Department of Psychiatry, THRIVE Gender and Sex Development Program, Nationwide Children's Hospital, Columbus, OH, USA

Department of Psychiatry, The Ohio State University College of Medicine, Columbus, OH, USA
e-mail: scottleibowitzmd@gmail.com

A. Janssen, S. Leibowitz (eds.), *Affirmative Mental Health Care for Transgender and Gender Diverse Youth*, https://doi.org/10.1007/978-3-319-78307-9_2

Gender Development

At this point in time, the field has not been able to pinpoint one specific factor that can explain how a given child or adolescent (or even adult) develops a particular gender identity. Gender identity development is thought to be multifactorial in etiology—biological, environmental, and cultural [1]—and there is no way to determine for a given person which factors are more influential than another.

In a rather useful review, Rosenthal provides an overview to the biological contributions to the development of gender identity [2]. In the review, studies that examine hormonal influences on gender identity are presented by looking at known entities where chromosomal, gonadal, and phenotypic sex are not aligned—of which there are many conditions encompassed by the larger umbrella term known as the "differences/disorders of sex development" (DSD), sometimes also referred to as intersex conditions. By studying women with pregnancies where babies who are XX with congenital adrenal hyperplasia (CAH) are detected on routine screening, researchers can measure the levels of in utero androgen exposure and track these infants over time. Ultimately, this has led to studies that quantify the effects of the degree of androgen exposure on future gender expression and gender identity [3–5]. Other conditions such as complete androgen insensitivity syndrome (CAIS) where the androgen receptor has a mutation that leads an XY infant to be born with female external genitalia (and thus reared as female) also demonstrate the possibility of a biological contribution to gender identity [6]. Describing the results of all the studies examining atypical hormone exposure to fetuses and the effects on gender identity goes beyond the scope of this chapter; however, one can make a case that there may be a biological contribution to gender identity development for a given person as a result of studies looking at hormone exposure to fetuses or children with sex diverse conditions.

Rosenthal also provides an overview of twin studies and brain imaging studies, which also demonstrate that gender identity development does have biological underpinnings. A review on neuroimaging studies in people with gender incongruence (another term for individuals who are transgender) demonstrated that brain phenotypes of individuals with gender dysphoria differ in various ways among sex dimorphic structures when compared to control groups of cisgender individuals, although the field is evolving and most of the studies done have included smaller numbers of individuals [7].

The prospective literature on childhood gender variance into adolescence is not vast, and that what does exist has limitations. There are only a handful of studies in the literature that follow prepubertal children into adolescence since 1987 [8–12]. A take-home message when these studies are cited in reference to understanding gender development of young children is that the majority of young gender diverse children do not display gender dysphoria after they begin to go through puberty. The research term for this is desistance. This has become a rather controversial discussion because the studies themselves vary in the populations they included and how they handled the children that were lost to follow up. The Green 1987 study focused primarily on gender nonconforming feminine boys and noted that only one out of the 66 boys studied was transgender in adolescence, with a large remainder of the boys later identifying as cisgender and gay. On the other hand, the later studies (most recently, the aforementioned Steensma et al., 2013 study) [10] demonstrate that the higher the intensity of gender dysphoria in childhood, the higher the likelihood for gender dysphoria to persist into adolescence. Limitations of all of these prospective studies include the fact that they did not use the current criteria for GD in the DSM 5. Previous iterations of the DSM (prior to DSM 5) were likely less accurate in capturing children who would meet the more strict criteria for GD of childhood as the criteria presently exist [13]. DSM 5 criteria for GD of childhood are explicit that a child must meet criterion A1 regardless of whether the child meets any other criteria, in order to have the diagnosis. Criterion A1 states: "A strong desire to be on the other gender or an insistence that one is the other gender (or some alternative gender different from one's assigned gender." Therefore, one could conclude that many of the children originally included in these studies were not transgender, per se, from the outset. From a diagnostic standpoint, stating that a majority of children with GD (DSM 5 criteria) are not likely to be transgender later on in life is inaccurate based on the change in criteria.

On the other hand, clinically and in the research, there are many children with significant prepubertal gender dysphoria (who may or may not have met the formal GD criteria in DSM 5) who ultimately do *not* experience gender dysphoria in adolescence. Additionally, the more recent research does in fact look beyond the criteria to measure the intensity of the feelings, which was correlated with persistence of gender dysphoria into adolescence, albeit without 100% predictive value. Therefore, the take-home conclusions of the prospective research of gender nonconformity in childhood that are reasonable to make would be: (1) the research has limitations as do all research studies; (2) this does not invalidate the research; (3) some children with gender dysphoria are no longer gender dysphoric once they go through puberty; (4) some children with gender dysphoria do experience worsening or persistent gender dysphoria once they go through puberty; (5) the more intense the gender dysphoria in childhood, the higher the likelihood of persistence into adolescence and beyond; (6) this is still not identified as a definitive predictor of persistence; and (7) there are no definitive predictors of persistence. In other words, we as clinicians have no definitive way to distinguish those children presenting with gender identity concerns who will be transgender later in life from those who will not. If the clinician believes the child will be transgender based on clinical impression alone, it still remains an educated guess. The point of emphasizing this is *not* to say that clinicians should *not* support children who identify as transgender, nor should they universally be against a particular intervention for those children; however, they (the clinicians) should simply be aware of this limitation that exists at this point in time, even when clinical impressions may lead them to believe otherwise.

Regarding adolescents presenting with gender dysphoria, research demonstrates that there is a much more definitive likelihood of persistence of gender dysphoria into adulthood. Three prospective studies from the Dutch VU Amsterdam Center for Gender Expertise demonstrate that adolescents who underwent a comprehensive psychodiagnostic assessment, received puberty suppression, and/or gender-affirming hormone therapy all moved forward with surgical gender transition, implying an unwavering gender dysphoria [14–16]. Qualitative data in a study on youth aged 10–13 years old indicated that this period was essential for them regarding whether or not they continued to experience gender dysphoria [17]. In this study, changes in social interactions with peers, emerging physical characteristics of puberty, and the first romantic experiences were identified as factors that influenced the youths' experience of their gender identity.

Indeed within the past decade, trends in clinical practice demonstrate changes that are important to take into consideration. First, the number of clinics in the United States has exponentially increased within the last decade [18] to approximately 40 as of 2014, with many more as of 2018. Additionally, as far as the prepubertal children go, parents are often deciding to move forward with a social gender transition for their child prior to ever seeing a mental health provider. There was a fourfold increase in the number of children presenting to the Amsterdam clinic having already socially transitioned to another gender from the year 2000 to 2010 [17]. Also, with respect to the adolescents, many more adolescents are seeking treatment for gender-related concerns than had in the past, and with new terminology and dimensional ways to think about gender (described in Chap. 1), research has yet to keep up with the evolving complexity. Understanding gender identity development from a research standpoint can often seem like a moving target as sociocultural shifts are made in society regarding the visibility of gender nonconformity and transgender individuals.

Yet these types of advances in understanding gender identity development, especially for those whose presenting with identities that differ from what would be expected based on assigned sex at birth, have significant clinical relevance. Families present to the mental health professional with different ideas about why their child may be expressing behaviors not stereotypically associated with their assigned sex. One parent may have an opinion that their child "is what their genitals say they are" and therefore the child could not possibly be a gender that is different from what they were assigned at birth. Another parent may view their child's behaviors as biologically wired and therefore see their child as transgender "who will always be transgender." Other parents may not know what to make of their child or adolescent's assertions and are confused, seeking the clinician's advice about who their child or adolescent is and how they should manage it. Without a blood test or brain scan at the disposal of the provider, we depend on our training as mental health professionals to navigate what might be complex clinical situations with sometimes profound ramifications.

Social Gender Transition

Defining Social Gender Transition

Social gender transition refers to the nonmedical process by which an individual lives as a different gender from that of the gender of their birth-assigned sex. This may involve the use of a different name, set of pronouns, clothing, and/or hairstyle depending on how stereotypical norms define gender for a particular culture. This may occur in some settings or in all settings and can occur at different paces for different individuals.

In Western society, gender is often thought of dichotomously based on binary sexes, which are typically separated into two distinct categories (male and female) throughout day-to-day life. Such examples of this throughout the environment include the presence of male and female bathrooms, two clothing sections in a department store, and implicit associations made between the presence of certain acceptable distinct behaviors/mannerisms for men (e.g., spreading legs when they sit) and women (e.g., wearing lipstick). In children, this dichotomy is reflected by associations between girl-ness and boy-ness and stereotypical activities (playing gentler for girls, playing roughly for boys), toy choices (dolls for girls, action figures for boys), and playmate preferences for children (historically children have been thought as "gender typical" when preferring to play with peers of the same gender). In adolescents, the gender binary impacts how youth might see themselves as they begin to experiment with romantic or sexual relationships, conforming to ideas about whom they *should* or *should not* have attractions toward, date, or engage in sexual behaviors with. These binary categories and constructs have been reinforced by popular culture and television that most children and adolescents are exposed to, whether it is in the mall, the school, or observations of people around them in public.

The DSM 5 uses language that shifted from a dichotomous categorization of gender (binary male and female categories) in previous iterations toward a dimensional understanding of gender identity and expression (gender along a spectrum) [13]. With this paradigm shift, in addition to a wave of sociocultural awareness of gender diversity, there has been a downstream effect on the way that clinicians think about the youth presenting in their office, often as some gender identity or expression that is different from the child or adolescent's birth-assigned gender (based on sex anatomy). Social gender transition now has multiple meanings. In the past, individuals thought of defining gender transition as a linear pathway from male to female or from female to male. Now, social gender transition can mean different things to different people. In addition to the previous traditional understanding of a linear and binary gender transition, it can now mean moving from one of the binary genders to living somewhere in the middle and staying put. It can mean moving between genders based on what authentically feels correct to someone at a given moment in time. It can mean moving to anywhere along a spectrum as a means of exploring what feels most correct for that person's identity within that person's environment. It may differ depending on the developmental stage of the child or adolescent. Their understanding of gender contextualizes the way they may live as a particular gender.

The degree to which a youth undergoes a social gender transition as a manifestation of a youth's already consolidated gender identity versus an exploration as to how it feels to live as a different gender can vary. The myriad of possibilities that exist regarding a social gender transition for a particular youth and family should be understood and considered as tools to not only address gender dysphoria for those youth who pursue social transition but also for those who do not necessarily meet criteria for gender dysphoria, yet desire to understand how living as a different gender may or may not affect their emotional and psychological functioning. Ethically, social gender transition—whether it be a manifestation of one's consolidated sense of self or an experimentation to discover what feels authentically correct—carries no irreversible effects on human physiology or anatomy. Additionally, there is no single definition of what social gender transition actually is, because sociocultural definitions of gender continue to change. Therefore understanding the concept of a transition for a particular person, which implies moving from one state to another, depends on how the states themselves are defined by that person.

Historical Approaches to Prepubertal Gender Diverse Children

Social gender transition in prepubertal children remains one of the more controversial debates in the field at present. There are different schools of thought, each with an emphasis on benefits and risks, yet there is no evidence-based treatment or consensus on how to approach the gender dysphoric child. Many an article or op-ed has suggested that there are "three approaches" to a child with gender-related concerns [19]. While these are reductionist ways of approaching a complex issue, it is important to summarize them simply as they have historically been described: (1) attempting to reduce gender dysphoria by increasing comfort with the child's behaviors and expression of gender associated with their birth-assigned gender; (2) "watchful waiting" by taking a neutral stance on gendered activities and expressions and not transitioning the child until they are older and might better understand the meaning of gender [20]; and (3) proceeding with an ego-syntonic social gender transition that provides the child the opportunity to live as the gender they assert, which is different from the one they are assigned at birth [21].

The approaches, as described, are rooted in philosophical beliefs about childhood gender development and whether it is influenced by external factors that could alter a particular outcome or whether it is an intrinsic innate characteristic that one is born with. The approach that has come under the greatest scrutiny and has even been considered to be akin to reparative therapy (a priori attempts to change an identity) is the first one listed above (attempt to reduce gender dysphoria behaviorally). It is important to emphasize that *any recommendations to redirect a child away from a behavior that is authentic and improves the child's sense of self and self-worth, yet might be considered "atypical" for the child's birth assigned gender, are considered harmful*. Such redirection runs the risk of promoting shame around activities and behaviors that can improve self-esteem, regardless of the child's identity at present or unknown identity in the future. Attempting to promote one outcome in the future (e.g., reducing the likelihood of the child having gender dysphoria in adolescence) through behavior modification leads the child to internalize messages about what is "right" and what is "wrong" for a boy or girl to do. Regardless of what the prospective literature states, suggesting that prepubertal children with gender-related concerns more likely to not experience gender dysphoria later in life, interventions that reinforce negative associations between behaviors and a particular gender could *still* have negative impacts on these children as well, even if they were to grow up and not identify as transgender. Therefore, the historically defined "active reduce gender dysphoria approach" would widely be considered unethical. If an element of that approach includes noncoercively increasing the repertoire of activities that the child is exposed to (e.g., exposing a boy who insists on being a girl to stereotypical "masculine" activities), so long as it does not *remove* the "feminine" activities that the child is naturally inclined to do, then that may be something for the clinician to suggest to the parents with the intention of breaking down the child's internalization of rigid binary gender role associations. The important thing to distinguish is the "adding activities" (noncoercively) versus "removing activities" element, with the latter being harmful.

The second historically defined approach, "wait and see method," also comes with challenges if applied universally to all children presenting with gender-related concerns. Children live in gendered societies so to deny this fact may seem to create an impossible reality for the child. And despite the fact that the etiology of gender dysphoria (either in childhood or adolescence or both) remains unknown, what is known is that a significant number of children will ultimately grow up to be transgender. Therefore to universally provide guidance that does not allow a child to socially transition (even without attempting to reduce their gender dysphoria), when in fact that may be a pathway to helping improve self-esteem and the opportunity to live authentically at a younger age, this approach, while cautious and not taking a stance in either direction, appears to be a unidimensional way of responding to a complex subject.

With the third historically defined approach, "support social transition," there are also challenges if applied universally to all children presenting with gender-related concerns. For the child who will ultimately persist with a transgender identity that remains stable throughout the rest of childhood and into adolescence and adulthood, the concept of socially transitioning earlier would appear to make sense so that they can live their most authentic sense of self from as early an age as possible. However, considering there are no definitive predictors of persistence of childhood gender dysphoria into adolescence, those with concerns about socially transitioning children at this young age is that it might "box in" a child into a pathway that otherwise might naturally would have subsided without the transition. For those children who do not necessarily feel boxed in and ultimately do not identify as transgender in early adolescence, a second gender transition that reverses to the gender of their birth assigned sex may be necessary. Anecdotally, parents who make the decision to transition their children at this young age may feel their own pressures from friends, family members, and society and therefore for some of them, tolerating the ambiguity of the future could be difficult, should the clinician raise the fact that their child might eventually reverse course.

A mental health provider or child and adolescent psychiatrist reading this section might wonder, "well if each of those three approaches have problems, how am I to assist a family presenting with a child who has these concerns?" The answer is to shift away from thinking about prioritizing a particular *gender identity outcome* (which are intrinsic to the philosophies and guidance behind each of these three historically described approaches) and to think about *emotional, psychological, and social functioning* of the child as the priority outcome measures. The concept of understanding each child on an individual level and guiding family decision-making in a nuanced way seems to be the most ethical approach to take [22]. As a point of opinion, reducing this discussion to "three treatment approaches" is problematic because it implies that as a clinician, one ascribes to one of three approaches, none of which have been systematically studied or has significant evidence to move forward with. Also problematic, is when one approach is labeled as "the affirmative approach" when in fact being affirming as a provider can mean many different things [23].

What does this all mean? To transition or not to transition, that is the question. Well, the answer lies in clinical judgment and the specific situation because children and families are complex systems and beings and no two situations are alike. The next section will focus on aspects of prepubertal social gender transition and will demonstrate that what is more important and relevant is about *how* the social gender transition is approached and managed (if approached at all) versus *whether or not* to transition the child.

Social Gender Transition in Prepubertal Children

Historical data on children who were gender nonconforming (meeting criteria for the predecessor category of GD in the DSM 5, gender identity disorder, a diagnosis that captures children who do not necessarily insist on being a different gender by today's standard) demonstrates that they are psychologically more vulnerable and more likely to demonstrate psychopathology of an internalized nature, such as depression or anxiety, versus externalizing behaviors [24]. Poor peer relations predicted the presence of psychopathology in those children; however, it is notable that this study published data on children who presented to one of two international gender clinics prior to the year 2000, long before the trend of prepubertal social gender transition increased. Newer research *has* demonstrated that prepubertal gender diverse children who socially transition demonstrate comparable (baseline) levels of anxiety and depression compared to age-matched controls (without gender identity concerns) and siblings at one point in time [25]. While this yields important information regarding the children, one cannot conclude from this research study that social gender transition is an effective intervention long term. Also, children who socially transition at younger ages are very likely to be supported by their parents who demonstrate love and acceptance. The parental support and acceptance as a factor itself could potentially mediate these low anxiety and depression outcomes, since the study did not compare these socially transitioned children to other gender diverse children who did not socially transition, yet might have had equally supportive and accepting families.

Table 2.1 Management aims when considering prepubertal social gender transition

• Enhance child flexibility and adaptive coping skills
• Help the child understand how others might respond to their expression of self in a non-pathological way
• Address co-occurring psychiatric or psychological issues and determine if those issues may be alleviated by a social gender transition or may be exacerbated by a gender transition
• Facilitate parental/caregiver acceptance
• Understand the motivations of the family to embark on a social gender transition
• Help family members understand their own experiences of rejection and/or acceptance to enhance a supportive connection with their child
• Consider a therapy referral for a struggling family member
• Understand the school and community climate and advocate to reduce bullying
• Advocate for the child across multiple systems that the child is exposed to: communities, faith-based institutions, extended family members
• Reinforce that all identity outcomes in the future may or may not happen as the child evolves and that they are both healthy and possible
• Intervene proactively in the event that harm is detected

Based on [22]

Not much direction on clinical management has been given since a review article was written by this author in 2012 [22]. Given how long it would take to capture long-term outcome data on the utility of a prepubertal social transition as an evidence-based intervention, it is important to approach each child and family individually. Therefore, a balanced, nuanced approach that is both affirmative of the child, yet appreciates both the benefits and challenges of a transition are important to factor into account. Therefore, the treatment management principles since the 2012 review article remain the same to date and are summarized in Table 2.1.

Some families may ask for assistance in how to best approach the social gender transition for their child. A clinician should consider all factors into the equation as determined in the gender-informed biopsychosocial assessment. First and foremost, a social gender transition should only be considered as a child-centered intervention. Therefore, the assessment should provide valuable information regarding how the child understands gender and the challenges that exist for the child by *not transitioning*, which are important aspects to guide decision-making. Sometimes a gradual transition, one that exists in the home or on vacation first, may be useful. This might give clues as to how the child responds to living in the gender role that they affirm at the time. This might start by using a different pronoun set or name and can then progress to more overt expressions of gender such as clothing choice and/or hairstyle. The clinician can also help provide psychoeducation on the unknown hypothetical benefits and limitations of pursuing a gender transition at this age, all within the context of the family dynamics and psychological profile of the child. The hypothetical benefits and limitations of pursuing a gender transition for this age group are illustrated in Table 2.2. Some families may wish to transition the child before a major transition (entering kindergarten or a new school) so that the child's assigned sex at birth can be kept hidden. This is referred to as living *stealth*. Some prepubertal

Table 2.2 Theoretical benefits and challenges of a social gender transition for a child with GD

Theoretical benefits	Theoretical challenges
• Affirms and supports a child's desire to live as a different gender • May eliminate co-occurring psychopathology when the untreated GD is determined to be a factor influencing the psychopathology • Allows a child who may be transgender in the future to live authentically from an earlier age	• May inadvertently "box in" a child who might not ultimately identify as transgender, depending on the child • Introduces the concept of going "stealth" (keeping it a secret), which may or may not be possible, depending on the child • Unknown challenges exist if a future reverse gender transition is desired

children are capable of living authentically and successfully in another gender without revealing their birth-assigned sex, while others may not (e.g., an impulsive child—say with ADHD—or a child who has difficulty negotiating healthy social relationships and prematurely trusts other children with sensitive information). While the concept of living stealth may seem preferential to families as a means of limiting the potential for bullying in school, an inadvertent consequence may be the shame-promoting message that it sends to the child in the event that it is not managed appropriately. For example, telling a child to keep this aspect of themself a "secret" can undermine the task at hand, which is to demonstrate love and support for the child and their gender diversity. Therefore, exploring the way this is communicated to the child as *private* versus *secret* may be beneficial so that the child does not internalize shame around the transition.

Sometimes complicated family situations can increase the complexity of the decision for the child to undergo a transition. In one situation, there may be parents who are fundamentally opposed to each other, and this might lead the child to perceive the discord between them to be around his or her gender. Therefore, it can be very difficult to determine whether the child is aiming to please one parent or the other. The intervention would be with the parents to help them realize that their discord itself may be a predominant factor in how the child presents. In another situation, a sibling of the child may have difficulty understanding what is happening in their family, and they may develop challenging behaviors that could put the gender diverse child at risk (e.g., acting out toward the child, announcing this to peers at school). Therefore, it is important for the clinician to be aware of all the possibilities about how the gender transition would affect the *family as a whole* and attempt to mitigate these negative effects through intervention, sometimes through anticipatory guidance or sometimes in reaction to what has already happened.

Clinicians must be prepared to manage clinical situations where a child has presented already having transitioned to another gender, sometimes initiated on their own, but more often occurring when their parent(s) are supportive of the notion of socially transitioning at this young age. Anecdotally, many of these supportive and accepting parents are presenting to the mental health provider with the purpose of establishing a connection so that when their child enters puberty, they have a mental health professional to advocate for next steps in their child's gender transition (e.g., medical transition). All too often, families and parents are planning for their child to receive puberty suppression (and even cross-gender hormone therapy after that) in several years' time, all with the best intentions of advocating for their child's mental and physical health. The child and adolescent psychiatrist or mental health clinician who read the earlier section in this chapter may recognize that this notion of a linear transition pathway that is core to the parental beliefs, itself runs counter to the fact that there are no definitive predictors of gender dysphoria persistence into adolescence, and therefore question whether that child would need those interventions later on. It is also equally important for the provider to recognize that the child *may in fact benefit* from these future medical interventions as well. An affirming provider will collaborate and develop trust with the parents/caregivers over time and become intimately familiar with the child and family, just as they would do with the "un-transitioned" gender diverse child, before determining that challenging the core beliefs held by the parents is appropriate. However, it may become important over time, for the provider to educate the parents that their child may ultimately identify in a different way (and perhaps not need pubertal suppression or other medical interventions). Helping the family convey a sense of openness and universal support for the child through interactions that convey the following overarching message: "We love you for who you are now, and we will support you no matter what, whether that changes in the future or not." This type of communication will help the child internalize the message that *all possibilities* are potential ones for them in the future and mitigates any negative concerns about parental imposition of a linear transition pathway on the child prematurely. This type of message also does not constantly increase the child's anxiety about their identity with repetitive inquisitions about who they are and statements that this might change in the future, which itself could be invalidating.

In summary, social gender transition in children is a rather complex subject, and there is no easy answer to guide clinicians. By focusing on positive emotional, psychological, and social outcomes, and determining the extent that a social gender transition can achieve those outcomes, the clinician can approach a complex subject with limited research and evidence-based directions and move forward with helping the child and family in an affirming way. A priori attempts to change a child's gender expression or promote a particular gender identity in the future are harmful. Lastly, thinking about the management of these children as ascribing to one of three approaches is overly reductionistic and does not take the individual and unique factors that each child and family presents with.

Social Gender Transition in Adolescents

Social gender transition in adolescents is less controversial than it is for children who are prepubertal. As noted, research studies have demonstrated that an adolescent with GD is more likely to experience GD long term. The social transition to another gender may be considered in two significant ways: (1) as a definitive step toward living in the authentic gender role that the adolescent experiences and/or (2) as an *exploration* to help the adolescent understand how it feels to be perceived in a gender role that feels most consistent with their internal experience. This distinction can be useful when working with the family as a whole, since parents/caregivers who are reluctant to acknowledge the existence of GD in their adolescent might benefit from perceiving the social transition as an *exploration* versus as a definitive path to a lifetime of medical treatments and/or surgical interventions. Often, the adolescent has been thinking about their gender for quite some time, yet their disclosure to their parents can occur much later. Therefore, the parents may need time to process the news. In some situations, the adolescent has been demonstrating gender nonconformity since childhood (which means that the declaration would be less likely to come as a surprise to the parent), whereas in others, the information might seem like an abrupt declaration.

As noted in Chap. 1 of this book, the use of pronouns and chosen name can be a first step for parents to use when managing the adolescent who desires to transition socially. Parents come to the pronoun and name discussion with a variety of ideas about what they represent. For some parents, the use of different pronouns means that they are automatically supporting a transition that includes hormones and surgeries, which many are fearful of. Others might be approaching pronouns with a genuine attempt to affirm the adolescent's wishes. Depending on multiple factors including the adolescent's temperament, coping strategies, level of rigidity or flexibility, and/or other co-occurring psychiatric presentations, an infinite number of permutations could exist when matched against parental beliefs, level of support, level of rejection, and ability to navigate their own fears about what the pronoun change might imply. The clinician can serve as a valuable conduit between the adolescent and their parent(s)/caregiver(s). Often, facilitating a pronoun change is a step that helps build trust between the adolescent and the provider. However, sometimes this may require shifting the frame of what the pronoun change might mean for the parent(s) or caregiver(s). In some situations, framing the pronoun shift as an "exploration" versus a definitive path toward the parents' biggest fear—*irreversible medical interventions*—can help them develop perspective on the issue. A doubting parent may think that the adolescent is "in a phase" and thus believe that switching to a different pronoun or name will automatically affirm an idea that they fundamentally do not buy into. Meeting the parent where they are at in terms of their belief will also build trust between the provider and the parent. Framing this in a practical manner to the effect of, "Let's see if you can try using a different set of pronouns and then see how your adolescent responds to that over a period of time." Then when meeting with the adolescent alone, helping them understand the way they express acknowledgment of the shift in their parents' *intentions* can be useful. These types of nuanced interactions often require the provider to be thinking on the spot and, in a way, acting as a negotiator to help bridge gaps where they exist.

Prioritizing safety at all times, it may be useful to help the adolescent feel comfortable exploring the gender role of their affirmed gender by suggesting they use clothing, breast pads and makeup (for the female-identified youth), or binders (for the male-identified youth) in the privacy of the clinician's office as a first step. Helping the adolescent detect which situations are safe or unsafe to be changing their gender expression to be more in accordance with their gender identity is a crucial aspect of this work. In some situations, there is a highly safe and supportive environment, yet a petrified adolescent. In this situation, working through the anxiety that the adolescent has would be primary. In other situations, the adolescent may be unnecessarily placing themselves into an unsafe behavior with limited capacity to detect the reactions of those around them. In that type of scenario, it would be important to help the adolescent understand how they might be perceived and develop better coping strategies that maximize their safety.

Embarking on a social gender transition in adolescence requires the clinician to be aware of these multiple aspects of the treatment framework: safety, resilience, individual coping, parent/caregiver support/acceptance, and school/community advocacy when appropriate. The gender-informed biopsychosocial assessment described in the previous chapter gives the provider the tools to manage these complexities and nuances.

As a social transition progresses, it is important to track the reduction or intensification of symptoms of other co-occurring psychiatric conditions that may exist. Understanding *why* the symptoms progress in the way that they do is equally as important, because they help frame the degree of benefit of the social transition itself. The following scenarios illustrate various possibilities:

> Vignette 1: Aiden is a 15-year-old birth-assigned female who prefers male pronouns and the name Aiden. He is depressed and wants his parents to use male pronouns and the name Aiden however they are skeptical that "this is a phase because he's just always depressed no matter what." He also is binding his chest to simulate a flat chest so he can be perceived of as male by strangers. As his parents increase their use of the pronouns after the clinician framed this as a useful way to help Aiden explore his gender (even though Aiden might not feel he is exploring), Aiden's depressive symptoms begin to abate. In session, Aiden notes that "feeling like everyone sees me as the true male I am is just an incredible feeling." His parents begin to realize that perhaps the improvement in depressive symptoms, in retrospect, are a result of his social gender transition.

This vignette is an illustration of the utility of a social gender transition to help parents experience their adolescent's happiness, which in turn may lead them to support the notion that their child is experiencing GD, and not as a passing phase. This demonstrates the dynamic changes that can occur by allowing different members of the family unit to experience the effects of an intervention over time.

> Vignette 2: Lily, a 16-year-old birth-assigned male, presents to her provider wishing to transition genders. This comes as a surprise to her parents who saw "no evidence of femininity at all in the past." Lily presents as highly anxious and tends to avoid conflict. She cares about her family's reactions because she knows they are well meaning. Her parents make every effort to use female pronouns, although they acknowledge how difficult it is for them. Lily's anxiety intensifies. Privately, her parents tell you, "We have been following your suggestions to use female pronouns but her anxiety is worse. Are you sure she really is transgender?" You meet with Lily privately and she notes that "I know this is my true self, I just cannot seem to bear the pain of burdening my parents in this way."

This vignette is also an illustration of the utility of a social gender transition intervention as a means of eliciting a family dynamic and another treatment goal that needs to be optimized. The parent may have a valid perspective, although they are interpreting intensified psychopathology (anxiety) to infer that gender dysphoria is not present. Therefore, prioritizing treatment of Lily's anxiety in the context of the pronoun shift would seem to make sense at this point in the treatment. Subsequent response to the anxiety treatment would then guide additional decision-making should Lily begin to thrive emotionally as her parents continue to affirm her identity.

Vignette 3: Sam (birth name Audriana) is a 15-year-old assigned female at birth who presents as gender nonbinary who wants the parents to use "they/them" pronouns. Sam purposefully chose a name that is gender nonspecific. Sam has a history of three suicide attempts, and recently has been online more learning about transgender people. Their parents are unclear about Sam's intentions because just one month ago Sam was presenting in dresses, and the month before Sam was refusing to go to school unless they could wear a bowtie exclusively. Sam is very insistent that their parents use gender neutral pronouns and insinuates that any form of misgendering will trigger self-injurious thoughts. Sam's parents privately believe that "We feel held hostage. It's so difficult using these gender neutral pronouns even though we are trying. We really think that our child is easily influenced by others and do not have a solid understanding of this whole thing." You urge Sam's parents to be more consistent with using gender neutral pronouns and to use the name Sam. Two months later, Sam presents stating "I prefer to wear dresses only and I like my birth name Audriana." Sam's depressive symptoms appear to have abated.

This vignette illustrates the benefits of helping parents recognize the utility of affirming the adolescent's wishes, which were completely reversible. The use of a different name or pronoun, as difficult as it may be for parents, does not necessarily indicate a path toward medical and surgical transition. It may even be useful for the purpose of establishing diagnostic clarity, which in this situation reflects a lack of a diagnosis for GD.

In all three of the vignettes, the parents were skeptical and the adolescent had some degree of psychopathology. The first two cases demonstrate different ways in which the adolescent responded to the pronoun affirmation (subsiding depression vs intensified anxiety); however, in both cases, the adolescent's gender dysphoria did not waiver. In the third case, the use of pronoun affirmation was an effective tool at reducing the adolescent's psychopathology, yet the gender dysphoria subsided. In summary, social gender transition is an intervention that can be used both as a means of helping an adolescent live their authentic sense of self *in addition to* potentially exploring gender for the adolescent who has a less developed sense of self. Recognizing the complex interplay of family dynamics, personality attributes of the adolescent, coping strategies, degree of suffering from gender dysphoria, and potential co-occurring psychopathology is a crucial task for the provider when considering how to approach social gender transition for adolescents.

Other Psychological Interventions

Supportive Psychotherapy

Supportive therapy can provide the avenue for which the adolescent can navigate aspects of their gender identity, gender expression, and sexual orientation. Within therapy, they may be able to explore relationships, intimacy, future fears, aspects of self-loathing due to being transgender (internalized transphobia), social support systems, and develop appropriate adaptive ego strengths. Sometimes, an adolescent with GD is unable to transition medically or surgically due to either financial limitations or lack of parental consent and/or acceptance. The power of the therapeutic relationship with an affirming mental health provider who can help support the adolescent in this situation can be invaluable and may often be life-saving.

In the American Academy of Child and Adolescent Psychiatry Practice Parameter [26], and American Psychological Association's guidelines [27], there are certain aims of therapy, which include (1) heightening an adolescent's ability to accurately detect any unsafe situations in the social environment, (2) understanding the benefits and risks of self-disclosure across varying contexts, (3) exploration of hypothetical reactions of loved ones to any physical changes that might take place when and if those are initiated, (4) understanding how one's gender identity intersects with other aspects of identity (racial, ethnic, cultural, religious identities, as examples), and (5) the development of healthy coping strategies in the presence of potential stigma and adversity. These aims can apply to children as well as adolescents. They can apply to individuals exploring their gender or to those whose identities are stable. They can apply to individuals who identify as binary categories of male or female, or to those who identify somewhere in the middle of the gender binary.

Supportive therapy may also sometimes not be needed during periods when the adolescent is thriving emotionally and psychologically. However, gender dysphoria and transition can be a process that takes place over many years, and therefore supporting these adolescents may sometimes mean that a youth may present with additional adjustment-related concerns during a subsequent phase of transition, despite what may have been a relative long period of stability. It is important to be able to reengage in treatment or increase the frequency of visits during these times, should they occur.

Psychopharmacology

There is no data or research to guide psychiatrists on psychopharmacological interventions and potential interactions with hormones and/or puberty suppression for adolescents with GD receiving those interventions. The overarching principle, as a child and adolescent psychiatrist would apply to any youth vis-à-vis the use of psychopharmacological interventions, would be to not initiate more than one intervention at a time. The task for the child adolescent when deciding on whether or not psychopharmacological interventions are appropriate at any given point in time for an adolescent with GD would be to determine the degree to which untreated GD is associated with the development of the psychopathology that the psychotropic medication would be used to address. This is not to say that both hormone intervention *and* an antidepressant would not be indicated, but what is important to discern would be whether or not the depression or anxiety is so impairing that it either clouds diagnostic certainty or impairs the ability for an adolescent to be able to handle the physical effects of the hormones in the event that they were initiated first.

Nonphysiological Transition Interventions with Psychological Benefit

The World Professional Association of Transgender Health, Standards of Care 7th edition (WPATH SOC7) also notes the following nonphysiological interventions to help GD in an adolescent [28]: (1) in-person and online support groups or organizations that provide social support and advocacy; (2) in-person and online resources for friends and family; (3) breast binding (for assigned females at birth) or padding (for assigned males at birth); (4) genital tucking, penile prostheses, or padding of the hips and buttocks; (5) name and gender marker changes in identity documents; (6) voice and communication therapy with a speech and language pathologist to develop both verbal and nonverbal communication skills that facilitate additional comfort with their gender identity; and (7) hair removal through electrolysis, laser treatment, or waxing.

Conclusion

Gender development, social gender transition, mental health care, and psychological interventions play a crucial development in promoting positive emotional, psychological, and social outcomes for children and adolescents across the gender spectrum. They serve as a means of both exploring gender when it may not be clear, but also in addressing co-occurring psychiatric symptoms that may be a manifestation of GD, independent of GD, or a symbiotic process with the challenges of GD. The role that the child psychiatrist or mental health professional has in the ongoing mental health treatment of these youth can be life-saving when the care is approached with nuance and the complexity is neither over nor understated depending on the individual clinical situation.

References

1. Steensma TD, Kreukels BP, de Vries AL, Cohen-Kettenis PT. Gender identity development in adolescence. Horm Behav. 2013;64:288–97.
2. Rosenthal S. Approach to the patient: transgender youth: endocrine considerations. J Clin Endocrinol Metab. 2014;99(12):4379–89.
3. Berenbaum SA, Bailey JM. Effects on gender identity of prenatal androgens and genital appearance: evidence from girls with con- genital adrenal hyperplasia. J Clin Endocrinol Metab. 2003;88:1102–6.
4. Dessens AB, Slijper FM, Drop SL. Gender dysphoria and gender change in chromosomal females with congenital adrenal hyperplasia. Arch Sex Behav. 2005;34:389–97.
5. Meyer-Bahlburg HF, Dolezal C, Baker SW, Ehrhardt AA, New MI. Gender development in women with congenital adrenal hyperplasia as a function of disorder severity. Arch Sex Behav. 2006;35:667–84.
6. T'Sjoen G, De Cuypere G, Monstrey S, Hoebeke P, Freedman FK, Appari M, et al. Male gender identity in complete androgen insensitivity syndrome. Arch Sex Behav. 2011;40:635–8.

7. Kreukels B, Guillamon A. Neuroimaging studies in people with gender incongruence. Int Rev Psychiatry. 2016;27(1):120–8.
8. Drummond KD, Bradley SJ, Peterson-Badali M, Zucker KJ. A follow-up study of girls with gender identity disorder. Dev Psychol. 2008;44:34–45.
9. Green R. The 'sissy boy syndrome' and the development of homosexuality. New Haven, CT: Yale University Press; 1987.
10. Steensma TD, McGuire JK, Kreukels BPC, Beekman AJ. Factors associated with desistence and persistence of childhood gender dysphoria: a quantitative follow-up study. J Am Acad Child Adolesc Psychiatry. 2013;52:582–90.
11. Wallien MSC, Cohen-Kettenis PT. Psychosexual outcome of gender-dysphoric children. J Am Acad Child Adolesc Psychiatry. 2008;47:1413–23.
12. Zucker KJ, Bradley SJ. Gender identity disorder and psychosexual problems in children and adolescents. New York: The Guilford Press; 1995.
13. American Psychiatric Association. Diagnostic and statistical manual of mental disorders. 5th ed. Arlington, VA: American Psychiatric Association; 2013.
14. Cohen-Kettenis PT, van Goozen SH. Sex reassignment of adolescent transsexuals: a follow-up study. J Am Acad Child Adolesc Psychiatry. 1997;36(2):263–71.
15. De Vries AL, McGuire JK, Steensma TD, Wagenaar EC, Doreleijers TA, Cohen-Kettenis PT. Young adult psychological outcome after puberty suppression and gender reassignment. Pediatrics. 2014;134(4):696–704. https://doi.org/10.1542/peds.2013-2958.
16. Smith YL, Van Goozen SH, Kuiper AJ, Cohen-Kettenis PT. Sex reassignment: outcomes and predictors of treatment for adolescent and adult transsexuals. Psychol Med. 2005;35(1):89–99.
17. Steensma TD, Biemond R, de Boer F, Cohen-Kettenis PT. Desisting and persisting gender dysphoria after childhood: a qualitative follow-up study. Clin Child Psychol Psychiatry. 2011;16:499–516.
18. Hsieh S, Leininger J. Resource list: clinical care programs for gender-nonconforming children and adolescents. Pediatr Ann. 2014;43(6):238–44. https://doi.org/10.3928/00904481-20140522-11.
19. Zucker KJ. On the "natural history" of gender identity disorder in children. J Am Acad Child Adolesc Psychiatry. 2008;47(12):1361–3.
20. De Vries ALC, Cohen-Kettenis PT. Clinical management of gender dysphoria in children and adolescents: the Dutch approach. J Homosex. 2012;59:301–20.
21. Ehrensaft D. From gender identity disorder to gender identity creativity: true gender self child therapy. J Homosex. 2012;59:337–56. https://doi.org/10.1080/00918369.2012.653303.
22. Leibowitz SF, Telingator C. Assessing gender identity concerns in children and adolescents: evaluation, treatments, and outcomes. Curr Psychiatry Rep. 2012;14:111–20.
23. Edwards-Leeper L, Leibowitz S, Sangganjanavanich V. Affirmative practice with transgender and gender nonconforming youth: expanding the model. J Psychol Sex Orientat Gender Diversity. 2016;3(2):165–72.
24. Cohen-Kettenis PT, Owen A, Kaijser VG, Bradley SJ, Zucker KJ. Demographic characteristics, social competence, and problem behavior in children with gender identity disorder: a cross-national, cross-clinic comparative analysis. J Abnorm Child Psychol. 2003;31:41–53.
25. Olson KR, Durwood L, DeMeules M, McLaughlin KA. Mental health of transgender children who are sup- ported in their identities. Pediatrics. 2016;137:e20153223. https://doi.org/10.1542/peds.2015-3223.
26. Adelson SL. Practice parameter on gay, lesbian, or bisexual sexual orientation, gender nonconformity, and gender discordance in children and adolescents. J Am Acad Child Adolesc Psychiatry. 2012;51:957–74.
27. American Psychological Association. Guidelines for psychological practice with transgender and gender nonconforming people. 2015. http://www.apa.org/practice/guidelines/transgender.pdf
28. Coleman E, Bockting W, Botzer M, Cohen-Kettenis P, DeCuypere G, Feldman J, et al. Standards of care for the health of transsexual, transgender, and gender-nonconforming people, version 7. Int J Transgenderism. 2011;13(4):165–232.

Chapter 3
Transgender Adolescents and the Gender-Affirming Interventions: Pubertal Suppression, Hormones, Surgery, and Other Pharmacological Interventions

Samantha M. Busa, Scott Leibowitz, and Aron Janssen

Introduction

> *I think I always just hoped that I would never get my period. I know I was in denial, but I still had this wish that perhaps it would skip me by.*

Prior to the beginning stages of puberty, apart from the genitalia, there is little that separates the phenotypic appearance of boys and girls. Prior to this stage of development, it truly is the clothes, hair, and demeanor that identify the boy or girl. For youth with gender dysphoria that intensifies or presents at the onset of puberty and adolescence, it is a time for identity consolidation as well as potential anxiety. It is at this time that the body begins to develop the secondary sex characteristics that differentiate men from women, and just like the teen quoted above, it is a time in which transgender youth must confront change in their bodies that may not be welcome. In this chapter, we will review the physiology of puberty and the medical and surgical interventions available for youth with gender dysphoria. Of note, the use of the term *medical* is in reference to those interventions that require prescriptions and are not provided by psychiatrists. It is important to clarify that psychiatric interventions, even if not exogenous in nature (e.g., psychological interventions),

S. M. Busa, PsyD (✉)
Department of Child and Adolescent Psychiatry, Hassenfeld Children's Hospital at NYU Langone, New York, NY, USA
e-mail: Samantha.Busa@nyumc.org

S. Leibowitz, MD
Department of Psychiatry, THRIVE Gender and Sex Development Program
Nationwide Children's Hospital, Columbus, OH, USA

Department of Psychiatry, The Ohio State University College of Medicine, Columbus, OH, USA

A. Janssen, MD
Department of Child and Adolescent Psychiatry, NYU Langone Health, NYU Child Study Center, New York, NY, USA

A. Janssen, S. Leibowitz (eds.), *Affirmative Mental Health Care for Transgender and Gender Diverse Youth*, https://doi.org/10.1007/978-3-319-78307-9_3

can also be considered *medical*; however, for the purposes of clarity, in this chapter, *medical* interventions refer to those interventions distinct from psychological or social interventions described in the previous chapter.

Pubertal Stages, Physical Changes, and Hormonal Changes

Puberty is a stage of life that can be both exciting and anxiety provoking for teens and parents alike and can be especially complicated for those who are gender non-conforming. It is referred to as the developmental stage in which secondary sexual characteristics appear, and children begin to confront changes in their body that differentiate men from women, physically and physiologically. For the youth experiencing gender dysphoria, this is compounded, as these changes may not be welcome and can introduce further confusion and frustration with their bodies. Changes in puberty are typically first noticed in birth-assigned females between 8 and 12 years of age and in birth-assigned males between 9 and 14 years of age, spanning a wide range of ages as well as maturity socially.

Physiologically, puberty begins when the hypothalamo-pituitary-gonadal axis is activated and there is pulsatile secretion of gonadotropin-releasing hormone (GnRH) by the hypothalamus. The secretion of GnRH stimulates the pituitary to release luteinizing hormone (LH) and follicle-stimulating hormone (FSH) by the pituitary, which in turn stimulates the ovaries and testicles to produce estrogens and androgens in both birth-assigned females and birth-assigned males, respectively. For birth-assigned females, FSH is responsible for developing follicles, which contain developing eggs, and also assists with the production of estrogen. For birth-assigned males, FSH stimulates the growth of seminiferous tubules ultimately leading to the production of sperm. LH is responsible for producing androgen male hormone in Leydig cells aiding growth of the seminiferous tubules. Birth-assigned females produce more estrogen and birth-assigned males produce more testosterone during this time. These hormones are increased within the bloodstream, triggering the physical and psychological changes that occur in puberty.

Physical changes are a consequence of the aforementioned physiological and hormonal changes occurring in the body. Adolescents of the two typical binary sexes experience *adrenarche*, the onset of androgen-dependent body changes, such as growth of axillary and pubic hair, body odor, and acne, and *pubarche*, the appearance of sexual hair. Birth-assigned females experience *thelarche*, the onset of breast development; *menarche*, the onset of menstruation; and weight changes. They also experience changes in their breasts. Both typical binary sexes also experience changes to their body shape, muscle content, and fat content. Birth-assigned males experience changes in their penis, scrotum, and an enlargement of testes. In addition, birth-assigned males will experience nocturnal emission, involuntary erection, and eventually will experience their first ejaculation. At this time, they are considered to be capable of procreation. Marshall and Tanner (1969, 1970) [1, 2] defined and mapped the stages of puberty as a means of a common language between multidisciplinary health providers to describe the physiological, biological, and psychosocial changes that occur during puberty. Tables 3.1 and 3.2 delineate the Tanner stages defined and changes to the external genitalia, pubic hair, and height of individuals in each Tanner stage.

At the onset of Tanner stage II, youth with gender dysphoria begin to experience changes that begin to differentiate their bodies in to binary "categories" that may or may not be congruent with their own gender identity. By definition of those who meet criteria for gender dysphoria, these changes might cause significant distress, as the development of these secondary sex characteristics does not match their gender identity. The ramifications may be significant, as we know that transgender adolescents are at higher risk for a number of challenges at home, school, and socially. Puberty impacts *all* adolescents from the moment they wake up, to when they get dressed in the morning and go to school, until they go to bed at night, and so for these youth in particular it is important to understand the effect that puberty has on their emotional, social, and psychological development.

Table 3.1 Natal male tanner stages

Stage	External genitalia	Pubic hair	Growth
I	Prepubertal	Prepubertal	5–6 cm/year
II	Enlargement of the scrotum and testes; scrotum skin reddens and changes in texture	Sparse growth of slightly pigmented hair at the base of the penis	5–6 cm/year
III	Enlargement of the penis, length and then width; further growth of testes	Darker coarser curlier hair spreading over the pubic area	7–8 cm/year
IV	Increased penis size, growth and development of glans, scrotum and testes enlarge, scrotum skin darkens	Hair continues to look more adult-like, though has not spread to thighs	10 cm/year
V	Adult genitalia	Adult hair in quantity and type	No further increase after 17 years

Table 3.2 Natal female tanner stages

Stage	Breast development	Pubic hair	Growth
I	Prepubertal	Prepubertal	5–6 cm/year
II	Breast bud stage with elevation of breast and papilla; enlargement of areola	Sparse growth of slightly pigmented hair along the labia	7–8 cm/year
III	Further enlargement of breast and areola; no separation of contour	Darker coarser curlier hair spreading over the pubic area	8 cm/year
IV	Areola and papilla from a secondary mound above the level of the breast	Hair continues to look more adult-like, though has not spread to thighs	7 cm/year
V	Mature stage: projection of papilla only, related to recession of areola	Adult hair in quantity and type	No further increase after 16 years

Clinical Vignette

A 13-year-old transgender male (born with female anatomical features) reported that puberty had greatly impacted his view of himself and increased his anxiety socially. He stated, "I get dressed… sometimes I don't wear a binder in the mornings, it's so uncomfortable, I have to wriggle into it because it's tighter. I then have to adjust my breasts because they're fairly large, and if I'm not careful they look weird. I also have to periodically duck into a bathroom and readjust my binder to make sure that my chest looks 'natural' like a cis guys chest would look. I go through my daily routine and then I get on the bus, to go to school, the bus I take takes me very close to my previous school where everyone knew me as female. When that happens I'm always very worried someone will see me and be like 'oh that's deadname, that's her, that is a girl.'" This individual was interested in beginning a medical intervention and sought out help from me to work closely with his family to explore these medical options.

In the following section, we will review the types of interventions and the decision-making process that goes along with these interventions.

Medical Interventions

There are a number of medical interventions that are recommended for adolescents with gender dysphoria, which depend on how far advanced in puberty the adolescent has progressed according to current standards of care and clinical guidelines [3, 4]. These interventions are used to delay or reverse the physiological and visible changes that occur in puberty. We classify these types of interventions on the physical body as reversible, partially reversible, and irreversible.

Reversible interventions include the use of puberty suppression medications, which delay the development of secondary sex characteristics in order to buy time for a younger adolescent to mature into older adolescents who can then assent for more irreversible interventions such as hormones. The puberty-suppressing medications include gonadotropin-releasing hormone analogues (GNRHa), which are more widely used for children with precocious puberty. Other reversible medications that can be used to inhibit the effects of puberty in a pubertal adolescent include spironolactone, which has androgen-blocking properties for birth-assigned males, and oral contraceptive pills (OCP), which is used as menstrual suppression in birth-assigned females. All of the reversible interventions, if discontinued, will then allow the adolescent's body to resume the functioning that had been blocked or inhibited as a result of their use. Partially reversible interventions include the use of sex hormones, specifically testosterone for birth-assigned females and estrogen for birth-assigned males. These hormones lead to the development of secondary sex characteristics of the sex associated with the adolescent's gender identity regardless of the sex at birth. Finally, irreversible interventions include a number of different types of surgery, which will be described later in the chapter. We will examine the history, evidence base, indications, and ethical dilemmas related to each of these interventions.

Puberty Suppression

Medical treatment for gender dysphoria has a relatively short history of use within the medical community. The Amsterdam Gender Clinic in The Netherlands has been at the forefront of puberty suppression treatment in the context of gender dysphoria. This group of clinicians and researchers developed a protocol for the clinical management and treatment of gender dysphoria [5] in adolescents. This protocol recommended the use of GnRHa, a form of puberty suppression medication beginning at 12 years of age, as a means of (1) giving adolescents time to explore their gender, (2) determining whether or not more irreversible interventions would be appropriate for long-term gender transition needs, (3) temporarily ameliorating the distress of gender dysphoria by suppressing the development of irreversible secondary sex characteristics, and (4) preventing the need for more invasive procedures later on, should the adolescent ultimately decide to proceed with gender transition (e.g., without breast development, one need not go through top surgery, a mastectomy).

GnRHa mimic the action of the body's natural GnRH, shutting down the feedback loop in the hypothalamus and pituitary gland. GnRHa stop LH hormone secretion, ultimately preventing testosterone secretion for natal males and estrogen levels for natal females. GNRHa effectively shut down the HPG axis and decrease testosterone and estrogen levels. During treatment, pediatric endocrinologists should monitor adolescents. GNRHa come in the form of intramuscular injections or surgically placed implants. The use of GNRHa has some potential risks of use including impact on fertility and bone mass. There is also little data on the long-term impacts of prolonged use of these puberty-suppressing hormones.

The Amsterdam protocol recommended that pubertal suppression is initiated after the child enters Tanner stage II of development in order to understand how the young adolescent reacts to the changes brought on by puberty, considering the prospective literature at the time indicated that many children with gender dysphoria would ultimately not experience gender dysphoria in adolescence [6]. This protocol stressed the importance of a comprehensive assessment and noted that the potential and actual side effects to pubertal suppression do not outweigh the benefits of GNRHa treatment in appropriately screened youth. The protocol also recommended the use of gender-affirming sex hormones as early as 16 years of age, and finally surgery, if desired at 18 years of age.

Since this initial protocol was described, a number of studies have demonstrated that puberty suppression has a number of advantages when treating gender dysphoria of adolescence [7, 8]. The pause on pubertal progression that leads to the suffering associated with gender dysphoria allows for further gender identity exploration and evaluation in a multidisciplinary setting over time. Current research has continued to demonstrate the benefits of puberty suppression. Prospective data indicates that after being treated with GNRHa and subsequent sex hormone treatment for gender dysphoria, adolescents have comparable psychological adjustment when compared to cisgender adolescent controls [9]. Some adolescents feel that they are able to be perceived as their true gender more effectively, ultimately leading to positive effects on psychosocial adjustment in young adulthood [10]. Cohen-Kettenis and colleagues [11] conducted a follow-up case study of an adolescent who had puberty suppression treatment at 13 years of age, testosterone treatment at 18 years of age, and finally sex reassignment surgery (also known as gender confirmation surgery) at 20 and 22 years of age. This follow-up evaluated psychological, medical, and physical side effects and long-term effects of puberty suppression. This individual reported no regrets about the treatment protocol and was functioning well psychologically, intellectually, and socially. The individual's metabolic and endocrine tests were all within normal limits, and there were no noted health difficulties. In addition to this case study, de Vries and colleagues [12] conducted a study of changes in adolescent behavioral and emotional health who received puberty suppression between 2000 and 2008. Results of this study indicated that adolescents treated with puberty suppression had decreased behavioral and emotional difficulties, though still experienced body dissatisfaction. Despite this, adolescents in this study experienced fewer depressive symptoms and overall improvement in general functioning. Feelings of anxiety and other mood symptoms (e.g., anger) remained the same however. Taken together, these studies indicate that the long-term psychological effects of puberty suppression may outweigh the negative potential side effects when treating gender dysphoria.

The criteria for use of hormone therapy have been defined by the WPATH [3] and the Endocrine Society Guidelines [4] and state that use of hormone-suppressing therapy is indicated when (1) there is a persistent and pervasive history of gender nonconformity or gender dysphoria; (2) the gender dysphoria emerged or worsened with the onset of puberty; (3) any co-occurring psychological, medical, or social difficulties that might interfere with treatment are addressed; and (4) the adolescent and family have given informed consent. These criteria can be assessed through a psychodiagnostic assessment with an expert in gender-affirming treatments. Expertise in gender development, as described by the 2017 Endocrine Society Guidelines [4], is defined thusly:

> "(1) training in child and adolescent developmental psychology and psychopathology, (2) competence in using the DSM and/or the ICD for diagnostic purposes, (3) the ability to make a distinction between GD/gender incongruence and conditions that have similar features (e.g., body dysmorphic disorder), (4) training in diagnosing psychiatric conditions, (5) the ability to undertake or refer for appropriate treatment, (6) the ability to psychosocially assess the person's understanding and social conditions that can impact gender-affirming hormone therapy, (7) a practice of regularly attending relevant professional meetings, and (8) knowledge of the criteria for puberty blocking and gender-affirming hormone treatment in adolescents."

Despite the fact that puberty blockers are generally considered reversible in nature, there are some concerns and potential risks that should be considered when considering GnRHa for an adolescent who meets criteria for gender dysphoria. The following risks have been described, but it is important to note that the long-term risks have not been fully demonstrated nor studied prospectively. Leibowitz and de Vries [13] summarize these hypothetical risks in a review article. They include the possibility of (1) disrupting the exploration of an individual's experience of the gender of their birth-assigned sex; (2) impacting brain development and processes mediated by sex hormones that affect cognitive development and affect regulation, in particular for young people with co-occurring neurodevelopmental disorders; (3) impacting bone development and the effect on bone mineral density and fracture risk; (4) limiting genitalia growth, particularly relevant for birth-assigned males, which has implications in the future should the youth want to pursue genital surgery given the fact that sufficient penile tissue is necessary for the typical penile inversion procedure when creating a neovagina; and (5) affecting long-term metabolic processes that are still as of yet unknown.

It is important to note that current research is evaluating some of these potential risks. One fMRI study looked at executive functioning in adolescents with gender dysphoria treated with GnRHa and found no significant changes in a planning task [14]. Of note, none of the youth included in this study had any significant co-occurring neurodevelopmental disorders such as attention deficit hyperactivity disorder or autism spectrum disorder. Additionally, preliminary research on the effects of GnRHa on bone health indicates mild reduction in bone mineral density [15], but the implications on fracture risk were not studied. Anecdotally, it is described that when pubertal suppression is used to buy time to explore these issues, families may view the intervention as one step on a linear pathway for gender transition, without necessarily appreciating the exploration aspect that the premise of using pubertal suppression was originally based on. Therefore, parents may not feel the need to bring their adolescents in for continued exploration of gender in a mental health setting and then several years later may show up again with expectations to begin what they perceive to be the next step in treatment for their adolescents: cross-gender hormone therapy. Youth, parents, and families may have co-occurring psychiatric conditions that go untreated as a result, considering there may be a false attribution of these co-occurring symptoms as a *manifestation of* gender dysphoria instead of a *co-occurring condition* that may or may not exist regardless of the adolescent's gender dysphoria.

Ethical debates around pubertal suppression also exist in terms of timing of initiation of GnRHa, duration of treatment, and fertility implications. The original Amsterdam protocol recommended use of GnRHa begin at no less than age 12, but many youth will enter puberty at ages much younger than that. For those youth, waiting until age 12 (more relevant for the birth-assigned females on average) could mean that many of the benefits of pubertal suppression would be missed considering these youth may be well into the later stages of puberty by that time. However, given the unknowns of how long one can safely suppress puberty medically during a time when an adolescent *is physiologically supposed to be going through puberty*, suppressing puberty at 10 years of age could then introduce additional complex questions down the road regarding the timing of the initiation of hormone treatment considering one does not know how safe or unsafe it is to suppress hormones for an extended period of time, however that is defined. In addition to the medical unknowns, there is no data on psychological outcomes of waiting to initiate puberty at age 16 (whether it is the puberty of the patient's birth-assigned sex due to an unlikely reversal of feelings or whether it is due to the puberty of the patient's affirmed gender due to continued gender dysphoria). While fertility itself is not impacted by the administration of GnRHa in the event that the GnRHa is discontinued (as the individual will continue to go through their natural puberty), should the adolescent wind up moving directly onto cross-sex hormone therapy, then this could very possibly render an adolescent unable to reproduce biologically since they never would go through their birth-assigned sex puberty sufficient enough to develop mature eggs or sperm. One additional logistical factor that is important to consider is whether or not GnRHa can be covered by insurance, as gender dysphoria is currently an off-label indication and the medication can be extremely expensive to obtain, if not covered [16]. In many situations, even if indicated, lack of access to these medications can prohibit their usage for an adolescent.

Therefore, ultimately multidisciplinary care is optimal when making individual decisions for specific youth, and in the event that a multidisciplinary team is not readily available to the mental health provider, seeking expert consultation on these issues from multidisciplinary gender clinic center providers would be prudent. As with all interventions addressing a health-related concern, weighing the risks and benefits of moving forward with the intervention versus not remains a complex yet important component of the risk-benefit analysis. Discussing the fertility implications, surgical implications, and hypothetical unknown effects with families is important. The purpose of describing these complexities is not to suggest universal withholding of these treatments but to help the provider appreciate the full degree of factors that need to be considered when assisting families and youth.

Reversible Androgen Blocking and Menstrual Suppression

In addition to GnRHa, there are other pharmacological interventions that can be used to suppress the effects of hormones released during puberty. These are discussed in more detail in Nahata, Chelvakumar, and Leibowitz [16]. They may be beneficial to use with adolescents who cannot access GnRHa for either lack of insurance coverage or parental consent reasons.

Spironolactone is an antiandrogen agent that can be used as an adjunctive therapy to GnRHa, cross-sex hormones, or as a stand-alone intervention. It is a potassium-sparing diuretic that also has antiandrogen properties, blocking the effects of testosterone on birth-assigned males. Hyperkalemia is a known side effect of these medications, so whoever is prescribing them would typically monitor potassium levels. When used in conjunction with estrogen in a transgender female adolescent, this medication may allow for lower doses of estrogen to be used in order to achieve similar degrees of feminization. Their effectiveness and safety have not been studied in adolescents with gender dysphoria; however anecdotally, they have been used clinically to help adolescents feel their gender dysphoria is being addressed medically [16].

Oral contraceptive pills can be used continuously in birth-assigned females to suppress menstruation, which can be a rather distressing monthly event for the birth-assigned female with gender dysphoria. There are many types of oral contraceptives that can be used to achieve menstrual suppression; however, they should be prescribed by providers who are familiar with the differences and can monitor the effects safely. Data on the use of these medications for other indications (not gender dysphoria) with adolescents has demonstrated efficacy [17]; however, limited evidence is available on the psychological effectiveness of these medications in the transgender adolescent population [16]. The mental health professional may consider collaborating with a pediatrician or adolescent medicine specialist regarding the use of menstrual suppression to alleviate the distress that menses may have on the psychological well-being of the transgender male patient with gender dysphoria.

Gender-Affirming Sex Hormone Therapy

Gender-affirming sex hormone therapy to treat gender dysphoria includes testosterone for birth-assigned females and estrogen for birth-assigned males. The use of these hormones allows the individual to develop secondary sex characteristics that aligns with their core gender identity. The interventions also reduce endogenous hormone levels. This further affirms the individual's gender identity and is shown to have positive benefits for those who have gender dysphoria. The use of both estrogen and testosterone will potentially impact an individual's emotions as they are essentially going through a second puberty if GnRha were not used or if they are going through puberty for the first time in the event that GnRHa were used. The use of estrogen in birth-assigned males will cause the adolescent to slowly develop breasts, soften their hair, redistribute fat to potentially widen hips, and potentially feminize the face. Feminizing hormone therapy also includes the use of androgen-reducing medications described in the section above, as these medications decrease testosterone activity and help to minimize the dosage of estrogen needed. Testosterone used in birth-assigned females will lead to muscle mass increases, a deepening of the voice, and development of facial hair over time. Tables 3.3 and 3.4

Table 3.3 Estrogen effects and time course [3]

Effect	Onset	Maximum effect
Body fat redistribution	3–6 months	2–5 years
Decreased muscle mass	3–6 months	1–2 years
Softening of skin/decreased oiliness	3–6 months	Unknown
Decreased libido	1–3 months	1–2 years
Decreased spontaneous erections	1–3 months	3–6 months
Male sexual dysfunction	Variable	Variable
Breast growth	3–6 months	2–3 years
Decreased testicular volume	3–6 months	2–3 years
Decreased sperm production	Variable	Variable
Thinning and slowed growth of body and facial hair	6–12 months	More than 3 years
Male pattern baldness	No regrowth, loss stops 1–3 months	1–2 years

Table 3.4 Testosterone effects and time course [3]

Effect	Onset	Maximum effect
Skin oiliness/acne	1–6 months	1–2 years
Facial/body hair growth	3–6 months	3–5 years
Scalp hair loss	>12 months	Variable
Increased muscle mass/strength	6–12 months	2–5 years
Body fat redistribution	3–6 months	2–5 years
Cessation of menses	2–6 months	n/a
Clitoral enlargement	3–6 months	1–2 years
Vaginal atrophy	3–6 months	1–2 years
Deepened voice	3–12 months	1–2 years

show the expected onset of these changes for both estrogen and testosterone as well as the time to expected maximum effect.

The WPATH Standards of Care describe criteria related to treatment initiation. The standards require that individuals must be able to demonstrate capacity to consent to the medication and that any co-occurring psychological/mental health challenges are well controlled. Adolescents also must demonstrate persistent gender dysphoria. These criteria can be assessed through a psychodiagnostic assessment with an expert in gender development, as defined earlier in the chapter. In terms of age of initiation of this intervention, some prior guidelines recommend the use of gender-affirming hormones at 16 [18], though others recommend starting earlier in mid-adolescence [19]. The age requirement can be flexible, though it is recommended that when able, families should work together to support the adolescent seeking this type of intervention. The most recent recommendations from the Endocrine Society state that adolescents younger than the age of 16 should be eligible for gender-affirming hormones and strongly recommend an expert multidisciplinary team of medical and mental health professionals be involved throughout this treatment [4].

The definition of "well-controlled" as it relates to psychiatric co-occurring conditions is also not extremely well defined in the WPATH Standards of Care. Acute psychiatric conditions such as the presence of acute suicidal ideations, a recent psychiatric hospitalization, psychosis, mania, and/or a notable change in the functioning of the individual might be considered "uncontrolled." Long-standing depression and/or anxiety may very well be a manifestation of the gender dysphoria classification itself, and so therefore these issues could be alleviated with hormone treatment. A key task of the mental health provider is to determine the *relationship* between the gender dysphoria and any co-occurring mental health conditions so that the sequence and timeliness of the treatment intervention are appropriate. The cases in the rest of this casebook will serve to illustrate these complexities and guide the mental health provider when developing a treatment plan that is collaborative and affirming in nature with parents and the youth. On one hand, co-occurring psychiatric conditions could very well complicate the diagnostic picture, and therefore treatment of those conditions would be indicated to achieve a degree of "well-controlledness." On the other hand, needless delay of hormone treatment could perpetuate some of the psychiatric symptoms of the co-occurring conditions, and therefore it is prudent to determine the relationship between the gender-related concerns and other issues when considering the hormone therapy.

In addition to considering the criteria that are recommended to start gender-affirming hormones, individuals and families also need to consider the medical risks of gender-affirming hormones. These are outlined in the WPATH Standards of Care [3] and the most recent Endocrine Society Guidelines [4]. Estrogen may lead to increased risk for venous thromboembolic disease, cardiovascular disease, changes in lipid levels, liver enzyme elevations, gallstones, type 2 diabetes, hypertension, and prolactinoma. Testosterone can have an increased risk of polycythemia, weight gain, worsening of lipid profiles, and elevations in liver enzymes. In addition to these medical risks studied in adults, there are limited long-term research on these treatments for adolescents. In addition, for individuals who are nonbinary in their gender identity, this decision-making process may become especially difficult (see chapter on nonbinary gender identities in adolescents for further discussion of these complexities). As with all medical interventions, treatment providers and families need to have informed meetings about the risks and benefits of these medications. Since these interventions are partially reversible, families will be involved in a collaborative decision-making process with multiple parties who may have differing priorities.

Surgery

Gender-confirming surgical procedures are often considered the last step in addressing symptoms of gender dysphoria; however, this is not always the case. For many, use of gender-affirming hormones may be sufficient to manage gender dysphoria; however, for many others, gender dysphoria will not resolve until one or more surgical interventions have been sought. In adolescents, the most common surgery that is becoming increasingly recommended worldwide before the age of 18 is top surgery, or a mastectomy, for transgender males or individuals who are transmasculine with gender dysphoria. Genital surgeries are typically reserved for when an individual is 18 years of age or older.

There are a number of studies identifying the benefits of these surgeries including sexual satisfaction (e.g., Klein and Gorzalka [20]), psychological outcomes (e.g., Gijs, van der Putten-Bierman, and De Cuypere [21]), etc. Despite this evidence, there are fewer studies that include adolescents, as recommendations in the past stated that individuals should to be at the age of majority in their respective country for surgeries with case-by-case exceptions [3]. Overall, methodological difficulties related to studying the impact of gender-confirming surgeries add additional complexity to decision-making as many of the studies are retrospective and some of the interventions (e.g., phalloplasty, the creation of a new penis) still have not yet been perfected to the point where a multitude of patients who would normally seek the intervention would do so considering its complication burden.

One difficulty in studying surgical interventions is directly related to the wide range of interventions available. Types of surgery include “top surgeries” and "bottom surgeries." The reason why these surgeries are referred to as "top surgery" and "bottom surgery" is because referring to the specific anatomical feature for an individual who is transgender (e.g., breast, instead of chest) can itself be very challenging to hear. Table 3.5 explains the different types of top and bottom surgeries. Top surgeries include surgeries that are related to the chest and include reconstructive chest surgery and breast augmentation. Bottom surgeries are used to alter genitals or internal reproductive organs.

Other types of surgeries are used to change cosmetic appearance (i.e., face, head, and neck procedures). An individual may choose to have one, none, or multiple surgeries to address their gender dysphoria and live a life that they would like to live. These interventions are complicated and costly, ranging from $5000 to $50,000 and beyond. Besides monetary considerations, there are a number of potential medical and health risks, both short and long term, that are associated with these interventions. Some or all of these costs may be covered through health insurance, as many insurance companies are starting to classify these surgeries as "medically necessary." It is also important to consider the cost of not having surgery, which could be high, as many transgender individuals may continue to experience negative ramifications in public and private situations without the surgical interventions.

In regard to criteria necessary to be eligible for surgical interventions, the WPATH [3] recommends that consent can be given at the age of majority depending on the country the individual resides. While this is the recommendation, there are exceptions to this rule, and at times, there are younger individuals who seek out this intervention. Regardless, one letter for chest surgery and two letters for genital surgery are required for these interventions. Letter writers must be well versed in the diagnosis of gender dysphoria, and best practices dictate that surgeons discuss the different techniques available to the patient, the advantages and disadvantages of each technique, the limitations of the techniques, and risks/complications associated with the techniques for that individual. Individual anatomy and health factors are often taken into account. This is known as the informed consent process in order

Table 3.5 Surgery types

Surgery type	Name of surgery	Use
Top	Breast augmentation	Used to increase size of breast
Top	Reconstructive chest surgery	Removal of breast tissue in order to create a male-contorted chest
Bottom	Orchiectomy	Removal of the testicles, which can also eliminate the need for testosterone blockers
Bottom	Penectomy	Removal of the penis
Bottom	Vaginoplasty	Creation of a vagina using the tissue of the shaft of the penis
Bottom	Metoidioplasty	Increase of clitoris or phallus length without the use of tissue grafts
Bottom	Phalloplasty	Creation of a penis and scrotoplasty is the creation of a scrotum

for the patient to have a realistic expectation of the outcomes of their surgery. Some recommendations state that individuals should live continuously in the gender role congruent with their gender identity and adolescent transgender male patients seeking chest surgery should wait until at least 1 year of testosterone treatment is completed according to the WPATH SOC [3]. Collaboration and communication with the surgeon, just as the mental health provider would do with the medical providers, ensure that the patients' unique needs are best addressed. This provides the surgeon with the opportunity to understand the adolescent's psychosocial factors when discussing potential interventions. This also provides the mental health provider with the opportunity to learn about the surgical procedures, pre-, peri-, and postoperative course, potential complications, and other necessary pieces of information about the procedure so that they can assist the patient and family through the process.

One evolving area of clinical practice and research is related to the adolescents with gender dysphoria whose core gender identity is gender nonbinary. Many of these adolescents are seeking chest surgery exclusively and do not want the masculinizing effects of testosterone. It is important to understand what the desires of the patient are and take these factors into account when making recommendations that involve anything that is irreversible. Overall, the guidelines are less clear and require more targeted research to evaluate risks and benefits.

Conclusion

The role of puberty suppression, gender-affirming hormones, and surgical interventions is extremely important in the evaluation, management, and treatment of transgender adolescents. While there is some emerging research, there is still a lack of full understanding of the impact of these interventions medically, psychologically, and psychosocially. de Vries and colleagues [9] conducted a longitudinal cohort study of 55 adolescents who met criteria for gender dysphoria assessed before the start of puberty-suppressing drugs, at the initiation of gender-affirming hormones, and 1 year after gender reassignment surgery. This study indicated improved psychological functioning over time, fewer behavioral and emotional problems after puberty suppression, and finally, gender dysphoria persisted until gender reassignment surgery. While there are some limitations to this study, medical interventions are demonstrated to have an important impact on mental health considerations for adolescents and their families, and further research and advocacy is needed.

References

1. Marshall WA, Tanner JM. Variations in pattern of pubertal changes in girls. Arch Dis Child. 1969;44(235):291.
2. Marshall WA, Tanner JM. Variations in the pattern of pubertal changes in boys. Arch Dis Child. 1970;45(239):13–23.

3. Coleman E, Bockting W, Botzer M, Cohen-Kettenis P, DeCuypere G, Feldman J, et al. Standards of care for the health of transsexual, transgender, and gender-nonconforming people, version 7. Int J Transgenderism. 2012;13(4):165–232.
4. Hembree WC, Cohen-Kettenis PT, Gooren L, Hannema SE, Meyer WJ, Murad MH, et al. Endocrine treatment of gender-dysphoric/gender-incongruent persons: an Endocrine Society Clinical Practice Guideline. J Clin Endocrinol Metab. 2017;102(11):3869–903. https://doi.org/10.1210/jc.2017-01658.
5. Delemarre-van de Waal HA, Cohen-Kettenis PT. Clinical management of gender identity disorder in adolescents: a protocol on psychological and paediatric endocrinology aspects. Eur J Endocrinol. 2006;155(Suppl 1):S131–7.
6. Steensma TD, Kreukels BP, de Vries AL, Cohen-Kettenis PT. Gender identity development in adolescence. Horm Behav. 2013;64:288–97.
7. Cohen-Kettenis PT, Delemarre-van de Waal HA, Gooren LJ. The treatment of adolescent transsexuals: changing insights. J Sex Med. 2008;5(8):1892–7.
8. Wren B. Early physical intervention for young people with atypical gender identity development. Clin Child Psychol Psychiatry. 2000;5(2):220–31.
9. de Vries AL, McGuire JK, Steensma TD, Wagenaar EC, Doreleijers TA, Cohen-Kettenis PT. Young adult psychological outcome after puberty suppression and gender reassignment. Pediatrics. 2014;134(4):696–704. https://doi.org/10.1542/peds.2013-2958.
10. Lawrence AA. Factors associated with satisfaction or regret following male-to-female sex reassignment surgery. Arch Sex Behav. 2003;32(4):299–315.
11. Cohen-Kettenis PT, Schagen SEE, Steensma TD, de Vries AL, Delemarre-van de Waal HA. Puberty suppression in a gender-dysphoric adolescent: a 22-year follow-up. Arch Sex Behav. 2011;40:843–7. https://doi.org/10.1007/s10508-011-9758-9.
12. de Vries AL, Steensma TD, Doreleijers TA, Cohen-Kettenis PT. Puberty suppression in adolescents with gender identity disorder: a prospective follow-up study. J Sex Med. 2011;8(8):2276–83.
13. Leibowitz S, de Vries AL. Gender dysphoria in adolescence. Int Rev Psychiatry. 2016;28(1):21–35.
14. Staphorsius AS, Kreukels BP, Cohen-Kettenis PT, Veltman DJ, Burke SM, Schagen SE, et al. Puberty suppression and executive functioning: an fMRI-study in adolescents with gender dysphoria. Psychoneuroendocrinology. 2015;56:190–9.
15. Klink D, Caris M, Heijboer A, van Trotsenburg M, Rotteveel J. Bone mass in young adulthood following gonadotropin-releasing hormone analog treatment and cross-sex hormone treatment in adolescents with gender dysphoria. J Clin Endocrinol Metab. 2015;100:E270–5.
16. Nahata L, Chelvakumar G, Leibowitz S. Gender-affirming pharmacological interventions for youth with gender dysphoria: when treatment guidelines are not enough. Ann Pharmacotherapy. 2017;51(11):1023–32.
17. Altshuler AL, Hillard PJ. Menstrual suppression for adolescents. Curr Opin Obstet Gynecol. 2014;26:323–31.
18. Hembree WC, Cohen-Kettenis P, Delemarre-van de Waal HA, Gooren LJ, Meyer WJIII, Spack NP, et al. Endocrine treatment of transsexual persons: an Endocrine Society clinical practice guideline. J Clin Endocrinol Metab. 2009;94(9):3132–54.
19. Steever J. Cross-gender hormone therapy in adolescents. Pediatr Ann. 2004;43(6):e138–44.
20. Klein C, Gorzalka BB. Continuing medical education: sexual functioning in transsexuals following hormone therapy and genital surgery: a review (CME). J Sex Med. 2009;6(11):2922–39.
21. Gijs L, van der Putten-Bierman E, De Cuypere G. Psychiatric comorbidity in adults with gender identity problems. In: Kreukels BPC, Steensma TD, de Vries AL, editors. Gender dysphoria and disorders of sex development: progress in care and knowledge. New York: Springer; 2014. p. 255–76.

Chapter 4
Gender Dysphoria and Family Dynamics and Culture: A Case Composite

Melissa MacNish

Introduction

At the time of intake, Mia was a 13-year-old Vietnamese-American natal male who identified as a transgender female. She was in the seventh grade in an urban public school in Boston where she had grown up since birth. She lived with her mother and father, Ann (38) and Jim (41), who have been married 16 years and both immigrated from Vietnam in their early 20s. Ann's mother and father also lived in the same household.

Mia was referred to me by the school psychologist, Dr. Smith, after a weeklong hospitalization for suicidal ideation and self-injurious behavior. Dr. Smith reported that Mia disclosed her female identity to him 3 months before the hospitalization and initially had experienced a decrease in her depression and anxiety after the disclosure. Dr. Smith had been seeing Mia for the past 6 months for symptoms of depression and anxiety. Mia had also been prescribed Zoloft around that time by her psychiatrist, Dr. Lee. Mia had previously seen an outpatient therapist at the age of 10 and 11 for behavioral issues and ADHD symptoms. It was at this time that Mia began seeing Dr. Lee, who prescribed her Adderall. Mia's gender dysphoria began increasing with the start of puberty, and the disclosure of a transgender identity began to cause a great deal of conflict in the family. Since Mia's disclosure there had been an increase in arguments in the family, and Mia's depression and anxiety that had decreased after initially disclosing her identity to Dr. Smith and starting on Zoloft had increased drastically. Leading up to her hospitalization, she had not been attending school, had had an increase in suicidal ideation, had been cutting multiple times daily, had been vacillating between isolating from her family and intense emotional outbursts toward her parents and grandparents.

M. MacNish, MA, LMHC
Licensed Mental Health, SAYFTEE, LLC,
Jamaica Plain, MA, USA
e-mail: melissa@sayftee.com

A. Janssen, S. Leibowitz (eds.), *Affirmative Mental Health Care for Transgender and Gender Diverse Youth*, https://doi.org/10.1007/978-3-319-78307-9_4

After the first session involving Mia and her mother, it became evident that it would be important to have a Vietnamese-speaking therapist as part of the treatment team, as her mother and the rest of her family did not speak fluent English. We were able to find a Vietnamese-speaking therapist, Ms. Naguyen, at a downtown community center where the family received their medical care. It was decided that Mia's mother would meet with Ms. Naguyen biweekly as Ms. Naguyen could conduct her sessions in Mia's mother's first language, Vietnamese, and Ann already had a trusted, established relationship with the clinics where Ms. Naguyen worked. The author would meet with Mia weekly, and, because the gender specialist did not speak Vietnamese and Ms. Naguyen did not have experience with working with families around this topic, Ms. Naguyen and the gender therapist did joint family sessions on a monthly basis. Ann made it very clear that her husband would not be involved in the treatment. She reported that he knew of the "gender issues" but was not supportive of them; hence, at first the family sessions included only Mia and her mother.

Clinical Relevance

This case composite highlights the importance of taking a culturally informed assessment of the family when working with a transgender adolescent. It also addresses the following questions: How much can a family's culture and intersecting identities impact their acceptance? How does a clinician work with a family around their rejecting behaviors that are clearly impacting a youth's mental health? How does the therapist know how much an adolescent's mental health struggles are separate from (or correlated with) the stigma associated with being transgender, the degree of a family's acceptance or rejection, or their gender dysphoria? And finally, why is it important to expand the scope of care when working with the transgender and/or non-binary population?

Brief Literature Review

When an adolescent identifies as transgender and desires to make a gender transition, this puts a unique stress on a family [1, 2] and can tend to amplify any family dynamics that may already exist. Parents as well as siblings and extended family must go through their own process of grieving [3], understanding their fears, learning about gender and transgender identities, and accepting to integrate the new gender identity into the family [2, 4, 5]. When you explore further a family's intersecting identities in regard to religion, ethnicity, education, class, race, and age, it can complicate their process even further [2, 6–8]. Transgender stigma exists on a "structural, interpersonal, and individual level" and is the fundamental cause of adverse health effects in the transgender population [9]. Transgender youth and families who experience other marginalized identities must also navigate the intersections of these identities and the "unique constraints of oppression" that exist [6, p. 400]. This makes it even more important to identify the resilience factors of a family that they can draw on to as they go through the process [6].

A family therapy approach in the clinical assessment when working with transgender youth is not only of utmost importance because of the high level of dependence youth have on their families [10, p. 229] but also because family acceptance is directly correlated to a youth's positive mental health as they transition to adulthood [5, 11–13]. The therapist needs to assess each individual family member's understanding of the continuums (sex assigned at birth, gender identity, gender expression, and sexuality) [4, 8], exposure to transgender identities, access to support, level of acceptance, and personal stressors while also gaining an understanding of the cultural background and attitudes toward gender in the family. The therapist might also work with a family member to help them gain an understanding of their own internal barriers that might be getting in the way of their ability to accept and support the transgender youth as well as their feelings of loss [3].

When first meeting with a family, it is important to engage in a collaborative process that focuses on the family's resourcefulness [14, p. 46]. Throughout the therapy process, it is important to take note of both overt behaviors of acceptance and rejection as well as pertinent microaggressions. The therapist can then draw attention to them and try to reinforce the accepting behaviors and shift the rejecting behaviors. Ryan's [11] research shows that if a family can shift their behaviors from highly rejecting to moderately rejecting, it can decrease the risk of suicide attempts from eight times as likely to twice as likely [11]. Families that can shift their behaviors from not at all accepting to a little accepting can move an LGBT youth's belief that they can be a happy LGBT adult from 35 to 59% [11].

Coolhart [10] offers an important assessment guide for working with transgender youth. She categorizes the assessment questions into the following sections: early awareness of gender and family context, parental/family attunement to a youth's affirmed gender, current gender expression, school context, sexual/relationship development, current intimate relationship, physical and mental health, support, and future plans and expectations. In addition to these sections, this author finds it helpful to tease apart the information from the psychosocial assessment into three areas: internal stressors (mental health, risk factors around suicidality and self-harm, self-esteem, internalized phobias, etc.), external stressors (including family dynamics and the level of family support, other relationships, school communities, religious communities, neighborhood, etc.), and gender dysphoria of the youth (level of discomfort a youth has with their gender identity as a whole as well as with different areas of their body) in order to determine the focus of the intervention.

Interventions focused on internal stressors could include helping a youth increase their coping skills for mental health struggles around depression, anxiety, self-harm, and/or suicidality and supportive therapy to help build adaptive ego strengths [17, p. 29]. A psychopharmacological referral and/or neuropsychological evaluation can be helpful to understand better and address any mental health struggles the youth may be experiencing. Individual therapy focused on empowerment and resilience building will be helpful in the years to come. Interventions focused on the external stressors could include family therapy focused on shifting parents toward more accepting behaviors. Support groups for the youth and parents can reduce the stigma associated with a gender transition or gender nonconforming identity [4, 15, 16]. Conferences, retreats, and camps focused on the family can help increase a family's comfort level with diverse gender populations and help normalize this identity for parents. Interventions around external stressors could include working with a youth's school to ensure their safety and even working with faith communities to be open and affirming. Interventions focused on the gender dysphoria could include social transition and/or medical transition [2, 10, 17].

Working with transgender youth presents a myriad of complexities, and it is important to work toward having the youth be supported in all aspects of their lives. The therapist must be prepared to make referrals and interventions to expand the scope of care as this process requires support on many relational levels that include not only individual and family interventions but community and systemic interventions as well [2, 4].

Diagnosis and Assessment

History of Presenting Concerns

Mia's gender identity had been the elephant in the room and a source of stress on the family since she was younger. It was clear from a very young age that Mia's mannerisms and preferences were more feminine, and the family was clear that they did not tolerate this feminine expression. Since Mia recently told her parents of her desire to transition both socially and medically, her family seemed to be in a constant state of crisis.

Relevant Psychiatric History

Mia's behavioral and social issues began when she was 5 when she started kindergarten. She was very shy and quiet at school and struggled socially. In middle school Mia would spend most of her time at lunch in the bathroom crying silently in the stall. At 12, Mia began self-harming as she began noticing changes in her body with the onset of puberty. She would use a paperclip to make deep scratches on her upper arm where her parents could not see it. When Mia was 13, she began cutting and having frequent thoughts of suicide and was hospitalized for a week. After the hospitalization Mia reported that she was no longer cutting or having thoughts of suicide, but Mia's depression and anxiety continued to be significant as she pushed her family to support her in making a social and medical gender transition, and experiencing their resistance, her symptoms intensified. While Mia had never previously made a suicide attempt, she struggled with passive thoughts of suicide during most of our work together.

Gender Development History

Mia reported that she has "always known she was a girl." Her mother recalls getting a call home from school in kindergarten because Mia kept lining up with the girls. Ann reported that when Mia got home from school that day, she yelled at her to never do that again and never told her husband that it happened. Again in the third grade, Mia took her mother's nail polish and painted her nails, when her father got home from work he yelled at her and made her take the nail polish off immediately. Mia has always wanted to grow her hair long, but her mother always insisted on cutting it short. When Mia came out to her parents 6 months ago, she "took it back" after 2 months of having her parents berating her and making it clear that her feminine expression would not be tolerated in their presence. Mia then told her parents that she was mistaken and that she was probably just a gay male. Mia's parents were relieved by this disclosure. Mia's father told her that he was proud of her for being able to finally accept she was a boy and not to worry that she was too young to know if she was gay or not. However, after about 2 months into this new disclosure, Mia began to isolate herself from the family and started cutting again. With the help of the school psychologist, Dr. Smith, she was able to come out to them again and explain that she took back her initial coming out as trans as a way to protect the family from the shame they were experiencing. It was around this time that the referral to this clinician was made.

Psychosocial Factors

Mia's parents immigrated from Vietnam after they married. They reported they came to America to make a better life for their children as many of their relatives had done. They lived in Chinatown in Boston, and although their nuclear family had their own apartment, they lived among many extended relatives who made up their entire support system. The family was lower middle class and often struggled to make their co-payments. Ann worked as a waitress in a family restaurant, and Jim worked as a programmer in a start-up company. Mia's family was not currently religious, but they were both raised in the Buddhist tradition.

Mental Status

Mia was of slight stature. She typically would wear jeans and a plain T-shirt. She would often tie a knot in her T-shirt to make it tighter when she got into my office and was out of sight of her mother. Mia's hair was short in the back and longer on top; it was straight and dark. There were days where Mia was very animated during sessions. She would often get up and walk around while she talked. When she walked she would swish her hips and sway her arms. Other days when Mia was feeling less hopeful and sad, she would curl up in her chair and make little eye contact and would often become tearful. On these days her affect was depressed, and her thought process was very hopeless about her potential to be seen as a female in the world. She would perseverate on her changing body and voice.

DSM 5 Diagnosis

Mia came in with the following DSM diagnoses: major depressive disorder, generalized anxiety, and ADHD. After initial assessment that included a detailed gender history, it was clear that Mia fit the criteria for gender dysphoria. She was taking Zoloft to help manage her depression and anxiety and Adderall for her ADHD.

Preliminary Biopsychosocial Formulation

After taking a detailed psychosocial assessment of Mia and her family, I sorted the information I obtained into the following three categories to help formulate the treatment plan (Fig. 4.1). Mia's internal stressors included depression, suicidal ideation, internalized transphobia, guilt, shame, loneliness, self-harm, and anxiety. The external stressors that were impacting Mia were her family's process and their rejecting behaviors and the potential loss of community because of the stigma of transgender identity and a supportive school counselor who was aware of Mia's identity but concerned because the school had never have a student transition gender. When assessing for gender dysphoria, it was clear that Mia wanted to be seen as a girl by the world. Her deepening voice, increase in body and facial hair, and broadening shoulders caused her to feel intense anxiety and suffering. Mia has always hated her penis. From a very young age, she has sat down to pee and reported that she just tries to pretend it's not there. She disclosed having thoughts of wanting to cut it off.

From this assessment this clinician hypothesized that because of the intensity of Mia's gender dysphoria, the main intervention would be getting her parents to a place where they could support her in a social and medical transition.

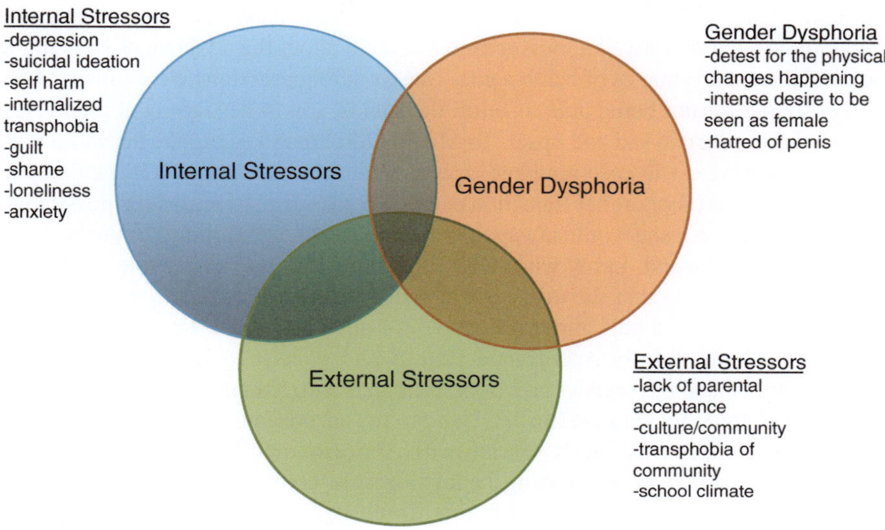

Fig. 4.1 Assessment sorting tool. This sorting tool can be helpful when trying to separate out the complicating factors when working with transgender youth in order to determine what intervention to focus on

Management

Treatment Course

In her work with Ann, Ms. Naguyen processed with her the many issues that come up for parents with transgender children (fears about the future, disclosing this to others, medical concerns, safety concerns, how this is a process for parents, etc.). Ms. Naguyen also discussed the many cultural concerns that Ann was struggling with. Part of Ann worried that Mia's mental health struggles were punishment from sins from a past life as she described the shame she felt from her child's psychiatric hospitalization. Ann also felt that Mia's gender nonconformity was disrespectful not only to Ann and her husband but Mia's grandparents and ancestors as well. Ann struggled to shift her belief that Mia was being selfish and bringing shame to the family name. Ann sorted through her feelings of losing her son and her identity as a mother with a son. As Ann grew to understand Mia's struggle and become more accepting, it became clear to Ann that she herself struggled with the limitations of gender expression within her culture and in the family. She started to become more empowered within herself as she began advocating for her child to her husband and to her parents.

In my work with Mia, it was clear that Mia was becoming more and more distressed as her parents were continuing to exhibit rejecting behaviors. Mia was secretly dressing in her mother's clothing, having passive thoughts of suicide, and sorting through intense feelings of guilt and shame. It became apparent that mom was sending both implicit and explicit messages to her child about the advantages of being a boy and the disadvantages of being a girl. These microaggressions were causing Mia to feel shame for not being able to fulfill the role of son in her family and guilt for making her mother so sad and upset. To Mia, it didn't really seem like her mom was making any progress in accepting her identity. When I would ask Mia if she thought her parents would support her transition eventually (as a tool to bridge the possibility of family rejection), she would always say to me that she was hoping for the best but preparing for the worst. In my work with Mia, I saw it as part of my role to prepare her for the possibility that she might not be able to transition until she was 18.

About a year and a half into our treatment, a shift happened. I was able to get a hard copy of the Family Acceptance Project and gave it to Ms. Naguyen. Ms. Naguyen translated the booklet and went through it with Ann in a session. Ann went home and shared this with her husband, and to my surprise he agreed to come in for a family session. In this family session with Ann, Jim, and Ms. Naguyen, we discussed how most of their rejecting behaviors were coming from a place of care because they knew how hard of a life this would be for their child. They believed that if they continued to discourage Mia's feminine expression and help her understand the disadvantages of being a woman that she would realize what a bad choice she was making. The therapists empathized with the parents' fears and validated them for trying to protect their child in the ways they knew how. The therapists tried to help Mia's parents understand that this was not a choice for her and referred back to Ryan's research at the Family Acceptance Project. The parents reported that they could tell that Mia seemed to be more sad and depressed when they discouraged her and made a commitment to not making so many negative comments to Mia.

I had been meeting with Mia for well over a year, and one of the things we had done together was to create her gender timeline. In a gender timeline, the client uses a large piece of paper on the wall and places their gender identity development and all of their gender-related memories onto a timeline from birth to the present. Mia spoke of her fears of transitioning (which were mostly around the fear of losing her family and her fears of not transitioning medically and having her body go through male puberty). In this session with both of her parents present, Mia presented her gender timeline. This clinician instructed her parents that they were not to interrupt and to listen to Mia's whole story. This clinician watched both parents fight back tears as they really listened to their child. When Mia was done, it was her dad that first spoke. He said, "I think I get it now. Your body and your heart do not match." Things continued to move in a positive direction after this session.

It was after this session that Ann agreed to take Mia shopping for some female clothes and both parents agreed to let her dress female at home. They also agreed to let Mia attend a weeklong summer camp for transgender children which they had refused to do the previous summer. Ann continued to refuse to go to support groups for parents with transgender children because she strongly felt that she would not be able to identify with the other parents. She felt that American parents were too permissive of their children and that they would not understand her struggles. Once Ann disclosed this as the source of her resistance, this clinician started a search for a Vietnamese-speaking parent of a transgender child.

Mia's experience at the camp was transforming. For the first time in her life, she was able to completely be herself and have that reflected back to her. Socially she did great and was even popular with the girls and was able to talk freely with her friends about the boys she had crushes on. When Mia came home from the camp, there was no stopping her; she was not going to wait until her parents got on the train; her train had already left the station.

Not long after the camp, one of my connections pulled through, and I arranged a phone call with Ann and another Vietnamese-American mother of a transgender child whose first language was also Vietnamese. I'm not sure if it was the camp, the phone call, or the combination and timing of both, but the family came in and said they were ready to make an appointment with the endocrinologist. They asked to start talking about how to make disclosures to family and what a social transition at school might look like. I contacted the safe schools program, and the school worked to train their staff and come up with a plan on how to support Mia when she started school in the fall as female. Mia met with an endocrinologist and started the process of hormone therapy. When Mia got home from the camp, she started attending a local support group for transgender and gender nonconforming teens.

Clinical Pearls and Pitfalls

When using this therapeutic assessment tool, the intention is to focus your therapeutic intervention on one area to see its effect on the other areas ideally decreasing the internal and external stressors and gender dysphoria (Fig. 4.2). Upon intake Mia's internal stressors, external stressors, and gender dysphoria were very high. The first

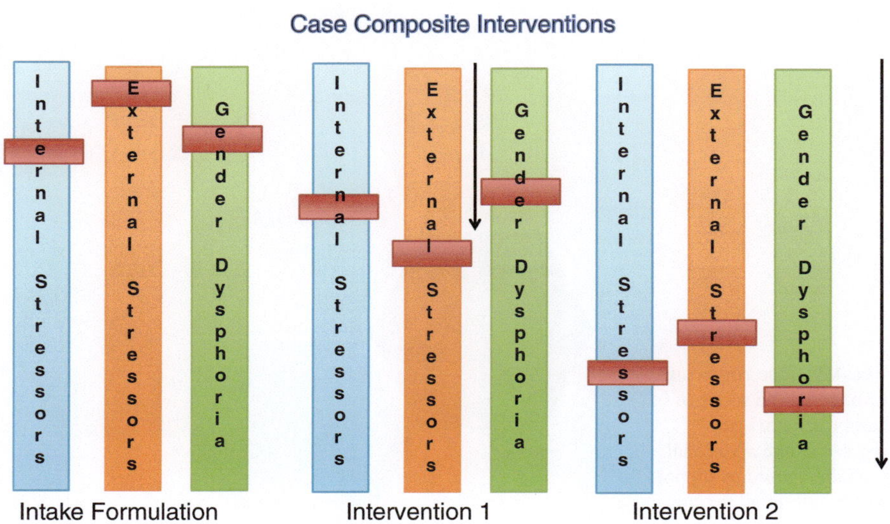

Fig. 4.2 Case composite interventions. Using the therapeutic assessment tool highlights the interventions

intervention focused on decreasing the eternal stressors, specifically the family dynamics. As the external stressors started to decrease, both the internal stressors and gender dysphoria decreased slightly. Once the external stressors decreased and the parents were more supportive, Mia was able to seek medical intervention. Once Mia was able to start socially transitioning, her gender dysphoria decreased significantly and in turn so did her internal stressors. The impact of this bidirectional relationship directly correlated with her external supports. As the scope of care was expanding, it helped to support the focus in treatment around the external stressors (Fig. 4.3).

This case composite highlights the importance of understanding a family's culture and how the intersecting identities of family members could potentially be a barrier to their acceptance of their transgender child. By using Ryan's research at the Family Acceptance Project with a family, a clinician can help them better understand the impact that their reactions and behaviors might be having on their child.

It can often be extremely overwhelming for a therapist to be faced with the task of assessing and supporting a transgender youth as they embark on a gender transition. Teasing apart the different realms internal stressors, external stressors, and gender dysphoria can help inform how much a youth's mental health struggles are separate from (or correlated with) the stigma associated with being transgender, the degree of family acceptance, and/or the degree of gender dysphoria. Expanding the scope of care is of utmost importance when supporting a youth and their family through a gender transition in order to support the youth in all three of these realms.

The most difficult challenge in this case for this clinician was bearing witness to Mia's suffering through the course of puberty as her body was developing in a way

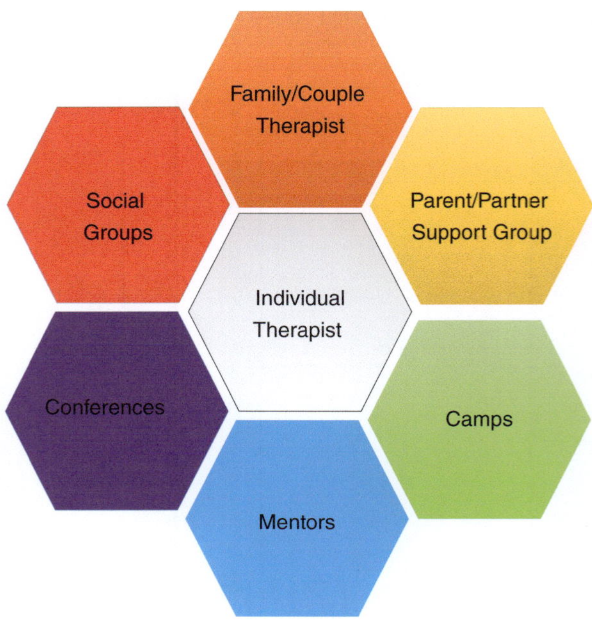

Fig. 4.3 Case composite. Expanding the scope of care. Each hexagon represents the additional modalities used to support Mia's individual therapy and well-being

that was intolerable to her. Puberty suppression was a possibility but only if Mia's parents would consent. Mia was very clear about her gender identity, but the process of therapy and moving forward with medical intervention could only go as fast as the parents' process would allow. It was almost 2 years from the time this clinician became involved in the case until her parents were ready to support her medical transition, it was already too late to stop the start of her puberty, and a lot of her secondary male sex characteristics had already begun.

Conclusion

This case highlights the need for a multifaceted approach when working with transgender youth. Often times much of the work is helping the family understand, support, and adjust to having a transgender child. A youth's identity can be impacted based on their parents' level of acceptance, as they often shape and reshape their lives for their children. Mia's identity as a transgender child forced Ann to examine her own identity as the mother of a son. Ann finally made space for her child to claim her identity because she worked hard to shift her identity from the mother of a son to that of a mother of a daughter. Luckily she had the resilience to do this for her child. In the father's profound shift, the mother was given permission to not have to choose between her husband and her child.

What we know is that the more clients have exposure to information around gender diversity through in-person experience of knowing someone, reading about the issue, or seeing a positive representation in the media, the more they are able to reflect the identities of trans people and support each other in healing. It is important for us as therapists working with this population to expand our scope of care and at times to take the role of advocate. Because of the stigma still associated with a transgender identity, acceptance not only becomes an intrapsychic issue for the individual but a family issue, a systemic issue, and ultimately an issue of oppression.

References

1. Brill S, Pepper R. The transgender child: a handbook for families and professionals. San Francisco: Cleis Press, Inc.; 2008.
2. Lev AI, Alie L. Transgender and gender nonconforming children and youth: developing culturally competent systems of care. In: Fisher SK, Poirier JM, Blau GM, editors. Improving emotional and behavioral outcomes for LGBT youth: a guide for professionals. Baltimore, MD: Brookes Publishing Company; 2012. p. 43–66.
3. Wahlig J. Losing the child they thought they had: therapeutic suggestions for an ambiguous loss perspective with parents of a transgender child. J GLBT Fam Stud. 2014;10:1–22.
4. MacNish M, Gold-Peifer M. Families in transition: supporting families of transgender youth. In: Nelson T, Winawer H, editors. Critical topics in family therapy. New York: Springer International Publishing; 2014. p. 119–29.

5. Giammattei SV. Beyond the binary: trans-negotiations in couple and family therapy. Fam Process. 2015;54(3):418–34.
6. Harvey RG, Stone FL. Queer youth in family therapy. Fam Process. 2015;54:396–417.
7. de Vries KM. Intersectional identities and conceptions of the self: the experience of transgender people. Symb Interact. 2012;35(1):49–67.
8. Sennott S, Smith T. Translating the sex and gender continuums in mental health: a transgeninist approach to client and clinician fears. J Gay Lesbian Ment Health. 2011;15:218–34.
9. Hughto JMW, Reisner SL, Pachankis JE. Transgender stigma and health: a critical review of stigma determinants, mechanisms, and interventions. J Soc Sci Med. 2015;147:222–31.
10. Coolhart D, Baker A, Farmer S, Malaney M, Shipman D. Therapy with transsexual youth and their families: a clinical tool for assessing youth's readiness for gender transition. J Marital Fam Ther. 2013;39(2):223–43.
11. Ryan C, Russell ST, Huebner D, Diaz R, Sanchez J. Family acceptance in adolescence and the health of lgbt young adults. J Child Adolesc Psychiatr Nurs. 2010;23(4):205–13.
12. Wren B. "I can accept my child is transsexual but if I ever see him in a dress I'll hit him": dilemmas in parenting a transgendered adolescent. Clin Child Psychol Psychiatry. 2002;7:377–97.
13. Grossman AH, D'Augelli AR, Howell T, Hubbard S. Parents' reactions to transgender youths' gender nonconforming expression and identity. J Gay Lesbian Soc Serv. 2005;18(1):3–16.
14. Madsen WC. Collaborative therapy with multi-stressed families. New York: NY Guilford Press; 2007.
15. Malpas J. Between pink and blue: a multi-dimensional family approach to gender nonconforming children and their parents. Fam Process. 2011;50(4):453–70.
16. Hill DB, Menvielle E. "You have to give them a place where they feel protected and safe and loved": the views of parents who have gender-variant children and adolescents. J LGBT Youth. 2009;6(2/3):243–71.
17. Leibowitz S, de Vries ALC. Gender dysphoria in adolescence. Int Rev Psychiatry. 2016;28(1):21–35.

Chapter 5
The Gender Nonbinary Adolescent

Valerie Tobin and Shane W. Gahn

Introduction

What follows are two case composites that illustrate the complex layers that present in any adolescent case, as well as specific concerns regarding evaluation for hormone treatment in gender nonbinary young people. We present a case in which the provider recommendation indicates that the adolescent is not, for several reasons, appropriate to move forward with hormone treatment and one in which the provider recommendation indicates that such intervention is appropriate for the adolescent.

When working with an adolescent who identifies as gender nonbinary, the following questions arise:

1. Does the gender nonbinary adolescent meet criteria for the DSM classification of Gender Dysphoria?
2. How does the clinician address youth presenting with a nonbinary gender identity who desires a specific phenotype when sex hormones have binary effects?
3. How does one rule out the possibility that the adolescent's gender nonbinary identity is not a sociopolitical statement against the gender binary versus a stable core sense of self as somewhere in the middle?

V. Tobin, MS, APN, PMHCNS-BC (✉)
Behavioral Health Services, Howard Brown Health,
Chicago, IL, USA

Robert Wood Johnson Future of Nursing Scholar,
Rush University College of Nursing,
Chicago, IL, USA
e-mail: valerie_tobin@rush.edu

S. W. Gahn, MS, APRN-CNP
Department of Psychiatry, Nationwide Children's Hospital,
THRIVE: Gender and Sex Development, Columbus, OH, USA

A. Janssen, S. Leibowitz (eds.), *Affirmative Mental Health Care for Transgender and Gender Diverse Youth*, https://doi.org/10.1007/978-3-319-78307-9_5

Gender Nonbinary Identities and Gender Dysphoria in Youth

In the 2015 US Transgender Survey (USTS), 80% of those who identified as gender nonbinary were assigned female at birth [1]. Recently, the sex ratio of those who seek gender-affirming medical care has reversed from previously higher numbers of those assigned male at birth presenting in treatment to those who are assigned female at birth [2]. This has raised concern that some assigned females at birth may be reacting to external or internalized misogyny rather than having a core male gender identity as a component of their authentic sense of selves.

Western society has long assumed two distinct and opposite sexes, with matching gender roles and identities. The conceptualization of a person with gender dysphoria has reflected this division, assuming that patients desired to transition from their assigned sex at birth, either male or female, to the "opposite" one. This is apparent in the changing language of gender incongruence. The term *transgender* as opposed to the older term, *transsexual*, signifies that not all want a linear "sex change," with both hormones and genital (sex) surgeries. This may be true especially for people who identify within the gender spectrum.

The latest USTS of 27,715 adults reflects the diverse nature of gender identity among transgender people [1]. Over one-third of their sample identified with a nonbinary gender identity, and 61% of these respondents were age 24 or under [1]. This equates to over 5000 respondents who were gender nonbinary-identified young adults, many of whom desired some gender-confirming physical interventions. Those with nonbinary gender identities have been integrated into indigenous communities throughout the world for centuries [3, 4]. Gender diverse adolescents are increasingly asking us to assist them in their journeys toward living authentically through hormone and/or surgical treatment.

The latest edition of the Diagnostic and Statistical Manual of Mental Disorders supports access of nonbinary people to medical services under the diagnosis of Gender Dysphoria. The current wording includes "the other gender or some alternative gender different from one's assigned gender" ([5], p. 452). Being in the exuberant state of adolescence, young clients are creating their own terms to describe their nonbinary experience. The respondents to the USTS used many words which include, "genderqueer," "agender," and "two-spirit," the latter term used among some Native Americans.

Since there is so much variety in these identities, best practice is often noted to ask adolescents to describe for themselves what a particular identifying term means to them. This assists in the evaluation, helps the adolescent to clarify their own experience of their gender, and supports rapport with the client by communicating respect for their individuality. Nonbinary young people may use the conventional pronouns of "he/him/his," "she/her/hers," "they/them/theirs"; however, some have declared comfort with using another pronoun set altogether, such as "ze/zir." This can often be confusing across generations, considering parents are often of the mindset that gender falls within the traditional binary sexes, and therefore pronouns that differ from the binary may be difficult for parents to embrace.

Most research assumes a binary gender identity [6], and unless the opportunity is available to make a different choice, data will continue to reflect a cultural bias toward two gender identities, reinforcing the belief that there are *no other choices.* Healthcare institutions reflect these beliefs through electronic health records and rooming arrangements [7]. Despite the lack of guidelines, gender nonbinary adolescents may ask for, and benefit from, a variety of hormonal treatment options, such as induced amenorrhea, blocking endogenous testosterone or estrogen, or the use of cross-sex hormones to develop secondary characteristics not consistent with the assigned sex at birth.

Sometimes adolescents may desire to have a phenotype that is not realistically possible with current care, and for this it will be important to consult with medical providers to determine what can be expected from safe hormone regimens that meet appropriate guidelines [8]. For example, some patients desire to control precisely which secondary sex characteristics will develop with the initiation of hormones, i.e., no change in face shape with either estrogen or testosterone, yet desire a change in the pitch of voice. Some of these concerns are manageable with other interventions such as shaving or electrolysis for unwanted body hair without the initiation of an exogenous hormone. It is important, therefore, to get specific information about what changes the adolescent desires with medical treatments and whether or not those expectations are realistic and address an accurate clinical picture of gender dysphoria.

It is also possible that some presenting adolescents who identify as gender nonbinary are reacting to negative experiences in their environments based on societal reinforcement of a gender binary, such as homophobia or misogyny. Youth reacting to external stimuli (gender role expectations, harassment) will likely benefit from therapy to address their role and ability to navigate authentic expression of self within the challenging environment. This might include interventions such as family therapy, advocacy with schools, and/or individual therapy to build resilience and find social support. That is not to negate that many gender nonbinary teens have an internal sense of self that *is* nonbinary *and* are experiencing harassment based on societal expectations of an assigned, and undesired, gender role. In fact, it is likely that they *have* experienced victimization [9]. The more gender nonconforming the youth is, the more they are at risk for abuse [10]. Due to such complexities, a thoughtful, collaborative, and compassionate evaluation is prudent, and often required, in multidisciplinary settings before initiating medical treatment.

Case Report: Kay

History of presenting concerns: Kay is a 15-year-old, white, native English-speaking, assigned female at birth who identifies as "not male or female, I don't have a word for it yet." Kay is a name chosen by the patient and used with father, sister, and therapist. Kay would like the provider to use this name and pronouns they/their/them. These will be used throughout this text in *italics* to denote singular form of a pronoun set that is typically used in the plural form. Kay has started using they/them/their pronouns with friends and at school. Kay was referred upon discharge from an adolescent psychiatric unit. Kay's father, Miles, has full custody of the patient and presented with Kay for assessment.

Diagnosis and Assessment

Psychiatric history: Kay has a history of anxiety and depression that Kay believes started in elementary school. Six weeks ago, Kay was hospitalized for suicidal ideation after Kay told *their* guidance counselor that they had a plan to kill themselves by hanging. Kay told the hospital that *they* did not want to live anymore because *they* felt "like a freak," which Kay explained as, *they* are not male or female, but "somewhere in the middle." Kay had never heard of a person who felt like *they* did, and online only found resource for people who wanted to be the "opposite sex." At the hospital, Kay was prescribed Lexapro and referred to a therapist and the local gender clinic for an evaluation, psychiatric treatment, and support. Kay has been seeing *their* therapist for 5 weeks and reported a good rapport. The therapist also provided Kay with some reputable online resources about gender.

At the time of assessment, Kay reported difficulty sleeping, irritability, and problems with focus in school. Kay reported episodes of being awake for three nights in a row writing songs. When *they* are writing these songs, a "muse" comes to *them,* whom they describe as a beautiful woman who inspires Kay. Kay says the muse talks to *them* at night often and sometimes in the day. Kay feels very energized during these writing sessions, sometimes calls friends to sing songs to them and talk to them about all of *their* music ideas. Kay stated that some friends will no longer take *their* calls early in the morning and perceived this as a betrayal of *their* friendships. These episodes had been intermittent throughout the previous 6 months. Suicidal ideation began approximately 1 year ago. Kay disclosed self-injury by cutting *themselves* for the past 8 months, which had decreased since the hospitalization.

Kay filled out a Mood Disorder Questionnaire to assess symptoms for bipolar disorder. Kay had seven symptoms, which indicated a high likelihood of the disorder. The anxiety instrument—SCARED—was not indicative of a current anxiety disorder.

Gender development history: Kay had always been "androgynous." Kay and *their* parents never fought about clothes and Kay recalls wearing clothing typically associated with feminine children in the west as a young child, but when *they* started choosing *their* own clothing, *they* chose to wear pants. Sometimes *they* reported enjoying wearing eyeliner. Kay's interests have always been varied—music, drawing, and reading. Kay's friends have been of all genders.

Kay explained *their* gender identity as, "I'm not male or female, I'm just me." Kay said *they* have "always" felt this way. Kay often went shirtless at home as a young child and remembers when *their* dad first told *them* that *they* should start wearing a shirt all the time. This was very embarrassing, and Kay started to avoid bathing because *they* did not want to see *their* breasts. This occurred at age 10 and menstruation subsequently started at age 12.

Kay reported that *they* do not have any negative feeling about their genitalia; however, *they* feel very uncomfortable with *their* chest and menstrual period. These, Kay feels, are what really remind Kay of *their* female sex and what *they* most want to change to increase congruence with *their* identity. Kay's menses are irregular. Kay had recently started wearing a binder outside the house and two jog bras inside because *they* do not like how it feels when *their* breasts move. *They* do not wear the chest binder for more than 8 hours at a time as doing so is not healthy, Kay learned from multiple sources.

"I tried to be a girl," Kay said. In middle school, wanting to conform, *they* wore stereotypically western feminine clothing and makeup daily, and waxed off the hair that grew on *their* face, but felt increasingly depressed as *they* denied the masculine part of *themself*. "I don't like tight clothes and that's what all the girls wear." Kay described *their* bra being snapped and boys commenting on *their* chest. "First, I was too small, then I was too large. I just want them [breasts] gone." Kay was unaware of *their* chest size, or how to measure it, and said that the sports bra bands had felt "kind of painful" recently.

Kay described *their* 13-year-old sister, Anne, as very feminine. Kay wished for a long time that Kay could "be a normal girl like Anne." Kay's paternal aunt, who is gay, suggested that maybe Kay is a butch lesbian, but Kay said, "I like guys too." Kay identified as "pansexual," describing this as being attracted to people regardless of their gender.

Kay presented as unsure if *they* want testosterone because "I don't want to look 100% like a guy either" and especially does not want to risk balding, a known effect of exogenous testosterone. When asked about how Kay would hypothetically feel about being perceived as male in the event that testosterone treatment were to masculinize *their* body such that society did not see *them* as being nonbinary, Kay said, "I wish I never had to think about gender again." Kay expressed sadness at not having been able to access puberty-blocking hormones in middle school, as *they* could have stopped *their* chest from growing. Kay reported a desire for chest reconstruction because "when people see my chest the first thing they think of is female and even a binder doesn't hide it." Kay denied a wish to be a parent in the future, and that *they* would "never breastfeed" even if *they* changed *their* mind.

Psychosocial history: Kay lives with *their* father, Miles, and sister in a middle-class neighborhood in a suburban area. *Their* father works in the computer industry and had been telecommuting since Kay's hospitalization. Gina, Kay's mother, works in a real estate office. Kay presented to this office during freshman year in a local public high school. Kay had all passing grades, until last year when *they* started to struggle in school, eventually missing multiple days at a time. At the time of presentation, *they* were failing two classes and working with the school to set up an Individual Education Plan.

Kay denied a history of abuse. Kay reported being teased for "looking like a boy" in elementary school and for chest size in middle school. Privately, Kay disclosed that *they* have had sex with eight adolescent partners, boys and girls, mostly girls, over the past year. Kay used to sneak out of the house to engage in sexual activities, but Miles discovered this about 2 months ago and put alarms on the doors and windows. Kay never told the hospital or *their* therapist about this because *they* were too embarrassed and "no one asked." Kay has had receptive vaginal penetrative sex with cisgender boys and reported usually using condoms, but not always. Kay was not on any prescription or over the counter birth control (as could be obtained in Kay's state of residence). Sometimes Kay would drink alcohol and smoke cannabis with these sexual partners, but had stopped since discharge from the hospital. Kay denied history of pregnancy and had never been tested for sexually transmitted infections. Kay continued to engage in "cybersex" with an online girlfriend Kay's age who lives in another state.

Kay's parents were divorced 4 years ago, when Kay's mother Gina abruptly left the family. Gina has a history of bipolar disorder and instability, which is why Miles has full custody of his daughters. Gina did not attend the assessment appointment because she was uncomfortable with Kay's declared gender identity and about meeting with a mental health provider.

Kay reported *their* strengths as being good at music, visual arts, and writing. "My English and band teachers love me." Kay reported having a good relationship with *their* father, sister, and father's family. *They* have had a few close friends since childhood.

Mental status exam: Kay's BMI is in the 90th percentile. Kay entered the session willingly and felt comfortable speaking to this provider both alone and with *their* father in the room. Miles showed appropriate concern for, and engagement with, Kay. Kay presented with long, loose hair and was dressed in an androgynous style, with jeans, large sweater, and plain black boots. There was noticeable facial hair around jaw line, and client was wearing eyeliner. Kay's clothing was appropriate for age and weather. Kay was cooperative to questions throughout the interview, with appropriate eye contact, and *they* responded appropriately to social cues. Kay's speech presented as loud, pressured, and rapid. Kay reported *their* mood as, "all over the place." *Their* affect was labile and thought process was linear and goal directed. *They* reported suicidal ideation twice per week and denied any plan or intent to follow through with the suicidal thoughts. *They* had self-injured by cutting about three times since discharge from the hospital, "but no one else knows that." *Their* thought content included auditory and visual hallucinations. *Their* insight and judgment were poor while the fund of knowledge was age appropriate.

Diagnoses: Kay met criteria for bipolar II disorder with evidence of hypomanic episodes prior to starting on SSRI and significant family history. Symptoms include up to 3 days with little to no sleep during which they had greater risk taking, i.e., sneaking out at night, engaging in alcohol and drug use, with eight sex partners by age 15, and currently goal-directed activity of writing songs, calling friends to the point of alienating them. They also reported auditory and visual hallucinations.

Kay also met criteria for gender dysphoria of adolescence and adulthood with more than 6 months of experiencing incongruence with assigned gender and current gender identity. Kay expressed a desire to rid themselves of secondary sex characteristics (chest development, menstruation) of assigned gender and to be treated as a different gender than assigned at birth. Kay expressed distress that led to functional impairment associated with the criteria met for gender dysphoria. The expressed congruence was not merely a result of a perceived cultural or societal advantage to being male.

Management

Given the genetic predisposition, current symptoms, and the high risk for suicide in people with bipolar disorder, the first priority in the management was to stabilize Kay's mood. In doing so, Kay would be better able to reflect on *their* experience and options for gender-confirming treatment. Initiation of GnRH analogues, i.e., "puberty blockers," would induce menopausal symptoms, offer little benefit at this stage of puberty (already well beyond Tanner 3), and be costly. However, by suppressing menses (a completely reversible intervention), one key aspect of the patient's distress from gender dysphoria would be addressed, which provided the additional benefit of protection against pregnancy. Kay was referred to a gynecologist who works with gender diverse individuals to discuss these options and to screen for polycystic ovarian syndrome (PCOS), as Kay had symptoms (mild hirsutism, irregular menses, mild obesity) that indicated this was a possible diagnosis. Kay and Miles were in agreement with this plan.

Counseling was provided about the following: (1) safer sex, both in person and online; (2) psychoeducation about bipolar disorder and available medication for treatment; (3) sleep hygiene; (4) exercise to support sleep, mood, and health; and (5) fitting chest undergarments correctly for which Miles agreed to purchase a measuring ribbon so that Kay could accomplish this privately. Recommendations for psychotherapy with Kay's current therapist included: continuing psychoeducation about bipolar disorder, self-care, family support, mood charting, and stress reduction, with a therapist who is experienced with gender diverse adolescents.

A letter with diagnoses was sent to the school in support of the IEP, focusing on needs related to bipolar disorder. Sensitivity to the gender component of care was discussed beforehand with both Kay and Miles, specifically regarding how much information needed to be disclosed to the school. A phone consult was made with Kay's therapist about the diagnoses and treatment suggestions. Kay was provided resources to support connections with other gender diverse youth and a referral was given for a local therapy group for gender diverse teens who are also struggling with mood or anxiety.

It was not recommended to move forward with hormonal intervention (testosterone) at this time for three primary reasons: (1) Kay is early in *their* process of identity consolidation, (2) *they* express ambivalence about testosterone treatment and its side effects, and (3) *they* are not emotionally stable enough such that the degree of sophistication in thinking about irreversible treatments is to be considered sufficient. Adolescents must be able to assent to their medical care, and this level of mental health instability complicates Kay's ability to do so. Kay would instead benefit from opportunities to further solidify their gender identity and explore medical options before starting partially or completely irreversible treatments, such as testosterone and surgery. This would ideally be included as a goal within individual therapy.

For any gender nonbinary adolescent seeking hormone interventions with binary effects, the importance of sophisticated thinking addresses the following dilemma: How can the adolescent navigate the possibility that others in the world may consistently perceive them to be *the opposite gender* when in fact that is *also* not an accurate of how they see themselves? Since sex hormone effects are binary, nonbinary adolescents with gender dysphoria may not develop a phenotype identical to their authentic sense of self if they choose to use cross sex hormones. The hormone effects will also influence how others perceive and interact with them. Nonbinary adolescents with gender dysphoria who are ready to start cross-sex hormones have considered these complex issues and, despite them, articulate that their experience of gender dysphoria will decrease once they develop some or all of the secondary sex characteristics of the "opposite" gender. This requires sophisticated thought and identity consolidation. In Kay's case, *they* simply did not articulate this type of thinking - whether that be the result of uncontrolled bipolar disorder, a poorly consolidated identity, other factors, or a combination thereof. This decision may change in the future, as Kay becomes better able to articulate *their* nonbinary place in a binary world. While chest surgery may be helpful for Kay in the future, there would be a risk of a recurrence of depressive episode for any surgery, and Kay has not yet been adequately treated for bipolar disorder which thus elevates the risk for a poor postoperative outcome. Often gender-confirming surgeries do not take place until adulthood, when it is presumed that identity consolidation has taken place. However, some older adolescents (with the consent of their parents), who have been consistent in their identity, understand the risks and benefits, and are able to assent, benefit from chest reconstruction surgery. On the spectrum of gender-related surgical interventions, chest masculinization surgery is not as invasive as the typical genital surgeries. It was recommended that Kay and *their* therapist continue to discuss the benefits and risks of surgery and how that would affect *them* emotionally and psychologically.

Case Report: Tonia

Diagnosis and Assessment

History of presenting concern: Tonia is a 16-year-old African American, native English-speaking, assigned male at birth who identified as a nonbinary, gender fluid person. She presented with her adoptive mother and father to psychiatric nurse practitioner to a multidisciplinary gender clinic for an outpatient psychiatric diagnostic assessment and subsequent appointments. She was referred by her primary care provider as the patient was seeking medical gender-affirming interventions, specifically estrogen to help feel "whole." Tonia and her parents were met with together and separately. Her parents denied desire or need to speak with the provider privately, noting that they were open with Tonia and shared both supportive stances and concerns with her when needed.

Tonia reported feeling most comfortable using female pronouns: she, her, and hers. She used the nonbinary pronouns of *they/them/their* for a brief period of time at age 13 but described that she/her/hers pronouns are easier for most people to understand and use. The patient used this name and pronoun set in all settings regardless of who she was with. Tonia is a chosen name that patient had been using since age 13. The name Tonia is an adaptation of her birth name and was chosen as homage to her past and her parent's choice of name for her. Her name was not legally changed so billing and records will continue to show her legal name until she chooses to legally change her name. The desire to proceed with a legal name change was unclear at the time of assessment.

Psychiatric history: Tonia had been treated since age 7 for attention deficit hyperactivity disorder (ADHD), combined type. She was prescribed long- and/or short-acting stimulants since age 7 with good control of symptoms and minimal, if any, side effects. She had no noted change in sleep or appetite when taking her medication, and adherence was reported to be 29 out of 30 days with an increase in hyperactivity and distractibility when medication was missed. She had never displayed dangerous impulsivity since starting stimulants.

Tonia had been in counseling intermittently since age 7 in various settings including an outpatient academic center and private practice. The goals of past treatment had focused on academic success, depressive and anxiety symptoms, and disruptive behaviors that were described as boisterous, intrusive, and fidgety, not dangerous, harmful, or aggressive. She had never had counseling that focused on gender and sexuality but stated that she felt safe and that she had developed a therapeutic alliance with her past counselors when she disclosed parts of her identity. Tonia had never been hospitalized psychiatrically and had no history of self-injury but did have passive suicidal ideations before recognizing and coming out as gender nonbinary.

She noted that she did have a passive death wish prior to realizing her gender identity. She described this as the "worst place I've ever been." She never had a suicidal plan or intent to kill herself.

Prior to the interview, Tonia completed electronic-based screening tools including PHQ9 and SCARED. Both tools scored low, with some symptoms of, but not suggestive of, depression and anxiety disorders. Her parents completed the PHQ9, SCARED, CMRS, and Vanderbilts which were congruent with the patient's report, not suggestive of mania at present nor in the past, and indicated well-controlled ADHD symptoms, with no oppositional defiant or conduct disorder.

Gender development history: Per her parents and Tonia, when she was in preschool and kindergarten, she had friends of different genders, often playing dress up as male, female, and nonhuman characters. Her parents recalled one instance in first grade where she became very frustrated and distraught because she had to cut her hair short per school policy. She stated that she would start dressing in the female uniforms if she could keep her hair. This was not honored by her parents and her behavior was reported as withdrawn for weeks after having to conform to the male requirements.

As she entered grade school, she had more male friends. The school she attended frequently separated youth by their assigned gender for activities and sports. She subsequently started taking on more typical westernized male roles in play and activities as well as appearance. This continued until age 10 when she started spending time almost exclusively with other female peers. She was found with cosmetics and garments belonging to her female peers at age 11 but denied using them, frequently stating her friends had forgotten them in her school bag. She later admitted to "studying how they worked" by using the cosmetics in private and trying on padded bras to simulate breasts. Around this time, she reported that she started shaving all of her body hair and tried to grow out the hair on her head. She stated that at that time she remembered feeling like she wasn't "all male" and that she had some feminine traits and interests. She wondered if she was supposed to be born a girl but never talked to anyone about this at that point.

At the end of that same year, she came out to her parents as pansexual. She reported that she first learned what pansexual was by accessing social media at school and by talking to her cousin. Her parents reported that at the time they didn't quite understand what pansexual meant but warned her that at her age, she was not to be having sexual contact with anyone and this would be punished if she was caught doing so. Approximately 1 month after coming out as pansexual, she told her parents that she had felt not "all male" since she could remember and recalled being very confused about cutting her hair in grade school when the girls didn't have to. She stated that she knew she wasn't like the other girls at that time but felt she could dress or look differently and carry on as she had been doing.

At the time of assessment, she reported not currently dating but identified as pansexual, panromantic, and monogamous. She defined this as being open to romance and sexual contact with anyone she may make a significant emotional connection with regardless of their anatomy, gender identity, or gender presentation but only in the context of a committed monogamous relationship. She had dated cisgender males and females in the past but had been sexually active with only one cisgender female girlfriend who she dated for 6 months, using condoms and birth control for protection. She had been screened for sexually transmitted infections during a routine physical at her primary care physician's office, and results were negative.

Her stated desire was to feel "whole" with "less obvious traits." When asked to elaborate what this meant, she attributed her physical size and shape to being masculine and that she has to do significant interventions to appear less male, which included meticulous shaving and hair care, stuffing her bra to simulate breast development, and being vigilant about the pitch, inflection, and volume of her voice. She noted that she had to look more feminine than was authentically her style so that people did not assume her to be male.

When asked to describe why she felt nonbinary and gender fluid best describe her, she described that on some days she felt more feminine in the comfort she has with emotionality, nurturance, and interest in typically female-associated western habits. She stated that on other days she felt more masculine and aggressive. She stated that she knew these are stereotypes but it's "truly a feeling within me that I'm neither, just more similar to one or the other depending on my spirit that day." She stated, "I definitely don't want to change down there," meaning her genitals, and views these as part of her gender nonbinary identity, not deriving distress from them and identifying sexual activity as pleasurable.

Tonia reported a desire to start estrogen as soon as possible and had done significant research online and with her school nurse to look up expected changes and how long they will take. She had identified that the only thing she does not want is to lose the ability to get erections, as she enjoys masturbation with her penis and penetrative sex. She noted being comfortable with the concept of not being necessarily fully perceived as female given her identity as somewhere in the middle of the gender binary, yet she was clearly able to articulate why the development of female secondary sex characteristics was more in line with her authentic identity. She stated that she is not concerned about the fertility effects that estrogen may have. Her parents endorsed that she had always been aware of her adoptive status and had always identified that she would adopt if she were to want children given her own positive experience of being an adoptee. She stated that she knew of the expensive, time-consuming aspects of adoption and that some people may not want to adopt to her in the future, considering her presenting outside of the gender binary, but that the "right kid who needs me may come along some day and then it will happen." The desire to adopt had never wavered according to her parents and had evolved as she became comfortable and communicative about her gender and sexuality.

When asked how she would deal with the possibility of losing sexual function or pleasure if she started estrogen, she said she would seek treatment as she knew of other penis-bodied people on estrogen who had successfully used erectile dysfunction medications and some who actually thought they would miss erections but found new ways to be sexual with their partners and themselves. She still hoped to maintain her penis's sexual function but acknowledged that she could not predict how her body will respond. She noted that the best change would be "curves" and hoped for some breast development as this would allow her to wear some of her favorite clothing that she felt uncomfortable in currently, given that it revealed the breast padding she reported often using in her tops. She reported not wanting breast implants and stated that she was nervous about any type of surgery.

Mental status exam: The patient did not have any medical diagnoses and was otherwise healthy, in 75th percentile of height and weight. Patient presented as well groomed, wearing medium length dark natural hair, typically female subtle makeup, clean shaven face with no facial stubble, a baggy black T-shirt with simulated breasts, fitted tight female style acid washed jeans, and slip-on unisex sandals. Clothing was appropriate for current weather and season and was clean. Her voice was deep and would likely be perceived as male. She sat with her legs open or crossed, often bouncing throughout the interview, and fidgeting with objects provided in office. This behavior reduced over the course of the interview. Her movements were otherwise normal. She was cooperative with questioning and divulged intimate details with shyness at times, yet was less restricted when separated from her parents. Her eye contact was appropriate and she attended to and used social cues appropriately. Her speech was normal rate, latency, and volume. Her mood appeared to be euthymic to anxious. Her thought process was linear yet distractible at times, associations were logical, and content was appropriate to the situation. Her fund of knowledge was appropriate for her age and her insight and judgment were good. She denied the presence of suicidal, self-injurious, and homicidal ideations.

Psychosocial history: Tonia was placed with her adoptive parents, who are Caucasian, at age 2 days as a healthy baby and was legally adopted by her adoptive mother and father at the age of 9 months. She has three older siblings who were also adopted and of various backgrounds and ethnicities, not biologically related to her. Of her siblings, two are sisters and one is a brother. She lived with her parents in a middle-class diverse suburb of a major city where she lived her whole life, but the family had moved to different homes during her childhood. Her siblings all lived in the same town with her oldest sister living between homes and often unreachable. Her parents both reported having advanced degrees and worked full time in Science, Technology, Engineering, and Math (STEM) fields. Her family was noted to be supportive even though they don't know other gender diverse people personally and were unsure how to best address these topics so they often avoided related conversations. Even though her parents were uninformed personally, they did offer to take her to LGBTQ events such as the annual Pride parade, a gender-focused youth group, and an art exhibition held at the local LGBTQ community center when she asked them. Her siblings all provided verbal support she could be whoever she felt inside and they would still love her. She expressed that this felt genuine coming from her "rainbow family," meaning of various races and ethnicities, and they've historically celebrated their differences.

She reported having close friends at school and in the neighborhood. She liked doing cosplay and often attended conventions wearing costumes as nonhuman characters, both male and female characters, and agender characters. She reported enjoying writing poetry and short stories. As an athlete, she has competed and won in local and regional events in track and field competing with and against male athletes.

At the time of presentation, she was a sophomore at an alternative public high school. The environment was noted to be relaxed and "supportive of all humans." She denied facing discrimination as everyone at her school is "unique" in some way. Her grades were reported to be As and Bs, as they were through elementary school, but there was a decline in academic performance during middle school as she was navigating social interactions and establishing her identity.

She identified her sense of humor and a "laid back" demeanor as strengths of hers. She identified her stressors and challenges as school, her oldest sister's mental health concerns, "[gender] dysphoria," and trying to make people understand and accept her identity. She had never had any legal or protective service involvement other than during adoption.

Her parents denied any emotional, physical, and sexual abuse and neglect in her past, and she also denied this when interviewed alone. She had experienced loss of a close friend to leukemia at age 13 and had experienced bullying by multiple peers during her seventh and eighth grade years, particularly around her gender nonconformity. This had stopped now that she entered a supportive high school that is known for its no-tolerance environment, accepting of all identities. Her community is diverse, but she still noted some people may "break their necks" by looking at her differently when she speaks because of her deep voice and taller/bigger frame while presenting with a more feminine appearance.

Diagnosis: Gender dysphoria in adolescents and adults. Tonia expressed an experience of a gender identity that is not congruent with her assigned gender for a period lasting at least 6 months (actually longer). She demonstrated a strong desire to be rid of and has made significant attempts to conceal her male secondary sex characteristics such as her deep voice and facial hair. Rather, she has attempted to simulate secondary sex characteristics typically associated with sex-assigned females. Tonia articulated that these physical changes would lessen her distress about her body and current gender expression, which is more stereotypically feminine than she prefers, so that she can override the automatic assumption that she is male due to her current features. Her distress associated with gender dysphoria was verbalized though her description of efforts exerted to appear less male. Her level of distress was likely less than expected because of her very welcome and open environment at home and school. It was suspected that she would have significant distress were she to be in a more homogenous environment. Her level of sophistication in her thinking indicated that she had consolidated her identity on numerous fronts and was mature enough to appreciate the concept that her sought intervention would alleviate her internal distress as a birth-assigned male, even in a society that reinforces the concept of two distinct genders, neither of which truly fit for her.

Management

The recommended interventions for total health and wellness at this point in time were limited as she was assessed to be doing very well socially, academically, and emotionally. She was well supported through her primary care provider's treatment of ADHD but was determined to possibly benefit from health maintenance from a gender-informed primary care provider who is more experienced with the unique health risks faced by transgender/gender nonconforming people. This was determined to be especially true in the event that hormone initiation was recommended. It was determined to be important for her to know risks with initiation of estrogen treatment. Tonia had demonstrated proficiency at seeking reputable information by reaching out to her school nurse and Internet resources. She was well informed and accepting of the potential risks of estrogen therapy, understanding it is a "binary" hormone that exerts effects consistent with typical female sexual characteristics despite the fact that she does not identify as "fully female."

Tonia had addressed the possibility of regret and provides examples of how she has coped with regret in healthy ways stating, "we can never know what exactly we want in the future, but we do our best now, hoping for the best while preparing for something less perfect with the information we have." She felt she would not regret the changes and stated so in a rather articulate way. Her parents also verbalized awareness of the risks and expectations after having consulted with a provider knowledgeable about hormones. They stated that they are supportive and in agreement with her desires. It was therefore determined that she would benefit from an educational appointment with a pediatric endocrinologist to discuss the use of estrogen and antiandrogen therapy. If parents were then able to provide informed consent, and Tonia informed assent after counseling with pediatric endocrinologist, she would then be recommended to proceed with estrogen therapy.

Clinical Pearls/Pitfalls

These adolescents represent two distinct nonbinary experiences. Both meet criteria for gender dysphoria of adolescence; however, the experiences diverge in terms of their (1) degree of how well-controlled the co-occurring psychiatric conditions were and (2) differing levels of understanding of the discrepancy between the unknown future effects of a binary hormone and how that would address the varying levels of distress from gender dysphoria uniquely faced by gender nonbinary adolescents. Therefore, clinical decision-making that is comprehensive and nuanced, yet affirming and collaborative in nature is important, especially given the lack of evidence-based treatment modalities when approaching adolescents with gender dysphoria who identify as gender nonbinary.

Kay is just beginning to understand *themself* and receive the support necessary for their mental health. While Kay also meets criteria for gender dysphoria diagnosis, *they* are not interested in testosterone treatment at this time. Kay may eventually benefit from chest reconstruction, but further stability and exploration is encouraged before making this permanent decision, particularly in light of the fact that it would be important for the treatment team and parents (who need to consent, depending on the state) to have a sense that Kay is able to fully appreciate the fact that the irreversible interventions *they* are seeking may not in fact lead society to perceive *them* as neither male nor female. It is also vital to have a solid plan for postoperative care, and an adolescent will usually rely on family for this. At this time, Kay is likely to benefit significantly from gender-affirming mental health providers who can offer individual, group, and family support for both *their* diagnosis of bipolar disorder and gender dysphoria. Deepening *their* understanding of societal reactions to gender diversity and *their* desire to live outside the binary, in the context of better-controlled psychiatric symptomatology, may or may not lead to a recommendation for an irreversible intervention with binary effects.

In contrast, Tonia demonstrates sophistication in her thinking as evidenced by the explanations she provides around the possibility of undesired outcomes, such as being perceived female rather than nonbinary. She has clear ability to weigh theoretical pros and cons of hormones that produce typically female characteristics and how this would impact her nonbinary perception by others and potentially affect her own identity. Her reconciliation is clear in her description of moving away from male, rather than moving toward female. She has considered her future self not only in appearance but in regard to many aspects of self such as being a parent and a sexual being. She has been able to navigate her place as an African American individual who grew up with Caucasian parents and has been able to integrate this component of identity into her overall state of being. This shows she has moved into more abstract cognitive capabilities even in context of her ADHD, understanding there is not a singular decision without risk. She doesn't express that hormones will fix any problems she has existing in a binary normative society and acknowledges new hurdles she may face as a result of the effects of hormones.

Tonia's identity development is multidimensional, and she is well informed, supported by her family, and shows insight into herself and the effects of the sought medical interventions. She meets criteria for gender dysphoria. Though she has some complexity to her history with adoption into a multiracial home and ADHD diagnosis, these in no way impair her ability to assent to treatment and show examples of her resilience and self-acceptance. Tonia will most likely benefit from gender-affirming partially irreversible medical treatment (hormone therapy) and some supportive mental health involvement with a gender-affirming provider, particularly since she remains on medication for ADHD.

Conclusion

With increased visibility of transgender people in society, and a shift to more dimensional understanding of gender, adolescents are increasingly presenting along a gender spectrum. These young nonbinary people often desire irreversible binary interventions to affirm their identity. Little is scientifically known about clinical outcomes in these individuals so it is necessary to clarify the presence of gender dysphoria and understand the biopsychosocial context in which the adolescent seeks such interventions in order to assure that proceeding with partially or fully irreversible interventions is in the adolescent's best interest. Considering the gender nonbinary adolescent may never achieve a phenotype or reaction from society that is in accordance with their authentic self, helping the adolescent recognize the personal impacts of these interventions on their bodies and how they fall within today's society is important.

Therefore, we hope these cases illustrate the importance of being both affirming and sufficiently cautious when assessing adolescents' abilities to assent for partially irreversible interventions, such as hormones, or irreversible interventions such as chest masculinization surgery. The clinician first must assess for the presence of gender dysphoria, have a general sense of the consolidation of identity, consider the sophistication in the adolescent's thought process, and understand whether or not the distress that they are experiencing by being perceived as their birth-assigned sex, by definition, comes from within and is not primarily driven by external motivators. By focusing on other domains of identity (social life, ethnic identity, racial identity, academic identity), the provider has indicators to understand the whole person as one with a solid sense of self and whether or not that person can navigate being perceived as a binary identity (hormone effects when provided safely are generally perceived as binary) yet possess an authentic nonbinary gender identity in a binary world. This is in contrast to many binary trans adolescents whose goal is to be definitively perceived as *the other* gender and blend into the binary society completely. The shared goal for binary and gender nonbinary trans individuals is better understood as *not* being perceived as their birth-assigned gender; however, the goals diverge in terms of the degree to which the two groups desire to be perceived as *the other* gender. As the field grows and more evidence sheds light on best practices, we must take these highly complex aspects of identity into account when approaching clinical decision-making with the gender nonbinary adolescents we serve.

References

1. James SE, Herman JL, Rankin S, Keisling M, Mottet L, Ana M. The report of the 2015 U.S. transgender survey. Washington, DC: National Center for Transgender Equality; 2016.
2. Aitken M, Steensma TD, Blanchard R, VanderLaan DP, Wood H, Fuentes A, et al. Evidence for an altered sex ratio in clinic-referred adolescents with gender dysphoria. J Sex Med. 2015;12(3):756–63. https://doi.org/10.1111/jsm.12817.
3. Frohard-Durlent H, Dobson S, Clark BA, Doull M, Saeqyc EM. "I would have preferred more options": accounting for nonbinary youth in health research. Nurs Inq. 2017;24:e12150. https://doi.org/10.1111/nin.12150.
4. Independent Lens. A map of gender-diverse cultures. 2015. http://www.pbs.org/independentlens/content/two-spirits_map-html/
5. American Psychiatric Association. Diagnostic and statistical manual of mental disorders. 5th ed. Arlington, VA: American Psychiatric Association; 2013.
6. Carrotte ER, Vella AM, Bowring AL, Douglass C, Hellard ME, Lim MSC. "I am yet to encounter any survey that actually reflects my life:" a qualitative study of inclusivity in sexual health research. Br Med J. 2016;16:86. https://doi.org/10.1186/s12874-016-0193-4.
7. Eliason M. The gender binary in nursing. Nurs Inq. 2017;24:e12176. https://doi.org/10.1111/nin.12176.
8. Hembree WC, Cohen-Kettenis P, Gooren LJ, Hannema SE, Meyer WJ, Murad MH, et al. Endocrine treatment of gender dysphoric/gender-incongruent persons: an Endocrine Society clinical practice guideline. J Clin Endocrinol Metab. 2017;102(11):1–35. https://doi.org/10.1210/jc.2017-01658.
9. Sterzing PR, Ratliff GA, Gartner RE, McGeough BL, Johnson KC. Social ecological correlates of polyvictimization among a national sample of transgender, genderqueer, and cisgender sexual minority adolescents. Child Abuse Neglect. 2017;67:1–12. https://doi.org/10.1016/j.chiabu.2017.02.017.
10. Roberts AL, Rosario M, Corliss HL, Koenen KC, Austin SB. Childhood gender nonconformity: a risk indicator for childhood abuse and posttraumatic stress in youth. Pediatrics. 2012;129(3):410–7. https://doi.org/10.1542/peds.2011-1804.

Chapter 6
"I'm Here to Get Taller and Because I Want to Be a Boy": A Case of Down-Turner Mosaicism in a Prepubescent Gender-Nonconforming Child

Diane Chen, Courtney A. Finlayson, Elizabeth Leeth, Elizabeth B. Yerkes, and Emilie K. Johnson

Introduction

Youth with differences/disorders of sex development (DSD) are congenital conditions in which development of chromosomal, gonadal, or phenotypic sex is atypical [1]. DSD encompass heterogeneous conditions that fall into three main categories

D. Chen, PhD (✉)
Division of Adolescent Medicine, Department of Child and Adolescent Psychiatry, Ann and Robert H. Lurie Children's Hospital of Chicago
Chicago, IL, USA

Department of Psychiatry and Behavioral Sciences, Northwestern University Feinberg School of Medicine, Chicago, IL, USA

Department of Pediatrics, Northwestern University Feinberg School of Medicine
Chicago, IL, USA
e-mail: dichen@luriechildrens.org

C. A. Finlayson, MD
Department of Pediatrics, Northwestern University Feinberg School of Medicine, Chicago, IL, USA

Division of Endocrinology, Northwestern University Feinberg School of Medicine, Chicago, IL, USA

Department of Pediatrics, Ann and Robert H. Lurie Children's Hospital of Chicago, Chicago, IL, USA

E. Leeth, MS, CGC
Departments of Pathology and Pediatrics, Ann and Robert H. Lurie Children's Hospital of Chicago, Chicago, IL, USA

E. B. Yerkes, MD · E. K. Johnson, MD, MPH
Division of Urology, Ann and Robert H. Lurie Children's Hospital of Chicago, Chicago, IL, USA

Departments of Urology and Surgery, Center for Healthcare Studies, Northwestern Feinberg School of Medicine
Chicago, IL, USA

A. Janssen, S. Leibowitz (eds.), *Affirmative Mental Health Care for Transgender and Gender Diverse Youth*, https://doi.org/10.1007/978-3-319-78307-9_6

(i.e., sex chromosome DSD, 46,XY DSD, and 46,XX DSD) on the basis of chromosomal constitution, gonadal pathology findings, and phenotypic features [1]. While DSD conditions are sometimes associated with gender-atypical/gender-nonconforming behavior starting in early childhood, in the majority of cases, gender nonconformity does not lead to gender dysphoria (GD)—that is, the *Diagnostic and Statistical Manual of Mental Disorders, Fifth Edition (DSM-5)* diagnosis capturing distress stemming from incongruence between birth-assigned sex and gender identity [2]. However, GD is observed more frequently among individuals with DSD conditions than in the general population, with specific rates varying as a function of syndrome, syndrome severity, and initial gender assignment [3]. Thus, clinical management of DSD often involves discussion of the possibility of GD with parents at the time of diagnosis; this is particularly true among patients presenting with genital ambiguity at birth for whom delaying gender assignment is recommended until genetic and endocrine work-up have been completed [1].

Among youth presenting with primary concerns for GD, however, clinical care does not routinely involve any genetic or endocrine testing to rule out a DSD condition. It is notable from our clinical experience that parents sometimes ask whether laboratory testing should be completed to screen for genetic or endocrine "causes" or "explanations" for gender nonconformity, particularly among prepubertal children who strongly assert a cross-gender identity from early childhood. As has been our practice within the Gender and Sex Development Program (GSDP) at the Ann & Robert H. Lurie Children's Hospital of Chicago (Lurie Children's) [4], which provides care for both gender-diverse (i.e., gender-nonconforming or transgender) and sex-diverse (i.e., individuals with DSD conditions) youth, the recommendation when these questions arise is *not* to pursue genetic or endocrine testing unless there is a specific physical indication for work-up (e.g., genital abnormality such as clitoral enlargement or penoscrotal transposition, delayed pubertal onset, short stature). The rationale provided to parents is that gender identity development is influenced by a multitude of biological and psychosocial factors [3], and the vast majority of individuals experiencing GD do not have a co-occurring DSD condition. Thus, unless there is physical indication for genetic or endocrine evaluation of sex chromosome genes and androgen exposure, laboratory testing may be both an unnecessary expense and unnecessarily invasive. Additionally, whether or not GD co-occurs with a DSD condition does not change the clinical approach to affirm a child's gender identity and support them to live as they feel most comfortable.

Here we present the case of a 6-year-old prepubescent gender-nonconforming birth-assigned female whose parents initially presented without their child for a single consultation session with our pediatric psychologist to discuss how best to respond to their child's gender nonconformity and support ongoing gender identity exploration. Later that year, the child, now 7 years old, was referred for an endocrine evaluation for short stature by the primary care pediatrician. This evaluation revealed an atypical karyotype (i.e., chromosome makeup), prompting additional medical evaluation and treatment. During this time, the child also became more insistent in asserting a male gender identity and parents returned to our psychologist with their child for a comprehensive psychological evaluation to help guide treatment recommendations for GD.

As *DSM-5* notes, most individuals with a DSD who develop GD will have already come to medical attention at an early age [2]; however, this case brings up the question of whether there is any utility to routinely pursue a genetic or endocrine work-up in cases in which GD is the primary presenting concern without physical indication for a co-occurring DSD diagnosis. In addition, as public awareness about gender diversity has increased in recent years, there has been growth in specialized clinics providing medical and mental health care to gender-nonconforming youth [5]. Many of these clinics are emerging within tertiary care pediatric hospitals that also provide multidisciplinary care for youth with DSD conditions. Some of these programs are integrated with the same specialists providing care for both gender and DSD patients, whereas other institutions have separate programs with distinct providers caring for each population of youth. Lurie Children's GSDP has an integrated program with the same group of specialists working within both the gender development and sex development arms of the program. This case illustrates the benefit of joint gender-DSD programs, particularly when caring for youth for whom there is co-occurrence of GD with a DSD condition.

Case Report

Sam, short for "Samantha" (a pseudonym), is a European-American birth-assigned female who was 6 years old at the time her parents initially sought consultation from our pediatric psychologist. Sam's mother and father presented alone for a single session to better understand Sam's gender development and learn how best to respond to their child's gender nonconformity. Specifically, parents shared that they had "considered the possibility that [Sam] is transgender" but "get confused" when she makes statements like, "I'm kind of a girl *and* a boy." Parents wanted to ensure they were doing everything they could to support Sam and promote ongoing gender exploration.

Developmentally, Sam was born late preterm at 36 weeks gestation, weighing 5 pounds, 12 ounces, and received speech and occupational therapy from 2½ to 5 years of age. Sam lived with her parents and 10-year-old sister in the suburbs of a large Midwestern city and was repeating kindergarten. Parents identified Sam's "small size" as the only reason they elected to have her repeat a grade, describing Sam as an "excellent" student. Sam was physically healthy, and parents denied any pediatrician concerns about growth at that time. With regard to psychiatric functioning, parents described Sam as a "generally happy kid" and denied concerns about emotional and behavioral functioning. Some separation anxiety was noted, but was not associated with significant clinical impairment.

Diagnosis and Assessment

With regard to gender development, parents described Sam as gender-nonconforming since she was a baby. As a toddler, Sam was observed heaving dolls out of her crib and was always drawn toward sports, toy weapons, and super hero action figures, which parents noted was dramatically different than the play preferences of Sam's older sister. During play, Sam exclusively took on masculine roles and predominately socialized with male peers. She was described as "superphysical," "hyper coordinated," and "physically strong" with "a lot of muscles." Sam had intermittently made statements about "feeling more like a boy" or "wanting to be a boy" since the age of 3 or 4 years old, and also has asked parents if and when she can "get a penis." For several years, parents had allowed Sam to choose her preferred clothing and hairstyle, and she has chosen to wear clothing from the boys' section, including boys' underwear and bathing suits/swim trunks, and groom her hair in a short, masculine haircut. Sam has been routinely mistaken for a boy in public by strangers, which parents noted has always made her "very happy." Parents denied that Sam had ever asked them to use masculine pronouns (i.e., he/him/his), nor had she insisted on using male restrooms, though Sam would use the male restroom if accompanied by father and the female restroom if accompanied by mother in public. Sam's gender nonconformity did not appear to affect her social functioning—she was reportedly well liked by peers with many friends in school, and parents denied any teasing or bullying on account of gender-nonconforming behaviors.

As previously highlighted, upon presentation for care, parents already had considered the possibility that their child was transgender. In his role as a school administrator, Sam's father had prior experience supporting a transgender student in pursuing social gender transition in the school setting. Parents posed specific questions regarding the likelihood that Sam would ultimately affirm a transgender identity, whether and when social gender transition should be considered, what options were available should Sam ultimately desire to change her body, and what they, as parents, could and should be doing to support her.

Our psychologist provided psychoeducation about what is known and unknown about trajectories of gender nonconformity [6], rates of persistence of GD among prepubertal gender-nonconforming children [7], factors associated with persistence of GD [8], and different theoretical approaches to clinical management of prepubertal gender-nonconforming youth [9–11], including a discussion of the lack of consensus regarding social gender transition as treatment for GD among prepubertal youth. The gender affirmative model [10, 12] guiding clinical practice within the gender development arm of GSDP [4] was discussed with Sam's parents. Central to the gender affirmative model is the understanding that gender variations are *not* disorders and that gender may be fluid and nonbinary [10, 12]. Specifically, gender-affirming care was described as supporting gender-diverse youth in living as they feel most comfortable taking into account the best interest of the child emotionally, socially, and psychologically, and promoting exploration of gender without presuming a fixed trajectory with regard to gender identity development. Our psychologist also shared our program's position that pursing social gender transition (or not) is a family decision given the current lack of research evidence supporting recommendations one way or the other. Parents were encouraged to follow Sam's lead and provide an environment that promotes discussion about diverse gender identities and expressions through developmentally appropriate children's books. Emphasis was placed on the importance of parental support in predicting positive psychosocial outcomes [13, 14], regardless of how Sam ultimately identifies with regard to gender identity. Parents were provided with resources for peer-based support, including the local Parents of Transgender Individuals support group that is affiliated with PFLAG (formerly known as Parents, Family, and Friends of Lesbians and Gays), as well as Pinwheels, a local play group for prepubertal gender-nonconforming children and their parents. Parents also received recommendations for books they might find helpful in supporting and accepting Sam's gender nonconformity [15, 16]. Finally, parents were offered the opportunity to bring Sam in for a comprehensive diagnostic evaluation in order to assess her understanding of gender identity and expression; however, given that Sam was not exhibiting problematic symptoms of behavioral or emotional disorders or distress related to gender nonconformity, further evaluation was not explicitly recommended. Parents were encouraged to monitor for changes in Sam's functioning that would indicate the need for further psychological evaluation, including change in emotional, behavioral, social, or academic functioning, or increased insistence on a cross-gender identity or worsening body dysphoria.

Parents elected to defer scheduling further sessions with our psychologist until additional needs arose, communicating that the consultation and psychoeducation were helpful and reassuring. Five months after the initial psychological consultation, Sam's mother reached out to share that Sam's pediatrician had recommended an evaluation for possible growth problems, with differential diagnoses including constitutional growth delay, idiopathic short stature, Turner syndrome, growth hormone deficiency, and chronic illness. Sam was seen for an endocrine consultation 1 month later and a full laboratory work-up and bone age assessment was recommended. Chromosome analysis identified a 45,X [12]/47,XY,+21 [8] chromosome complement, meaning that in the 20 cells tested, 12 cells had 45,X chromosomes and 8 cells had 47,XY,+21 chromosomes. Subsequent independent fluorescence in situ hybridization (FISH) studies confirmed these results. Interpretation was reported as consistent with X/XY and trisomy 21 mosaicism. The consulting endocrinologist provided chromosome results to parents by phone, explaining that the resulting karyotype could be Turner syndrome or gonadal dysgenesis, in addition to Down mosaicism, and recommended pelvic ultrasound to examine internal organs and referral to the sex development arm of Lurie Children's GSDP. Eight months after parents' initial consultation with our psychologist, Sam and her parents were seen in our multidisciplinary sex development clinic by specialists from endocrinology, urology, psychology, and genetics. Of note, the psychologist family saw in clinic was the same psychologist with whom parents had their initial consultation.

Sam, now 7 years old, presented as a happy, friendly prepubertal child who was small for her age. Her hair was neatly groomed in a short, masculine haircut, and her clothing and glasses were consistent with masculine gender expression. Based on Sam's physical appearance, it was easy to understand why strangers frequently assumed she was a boy. Sam's understanding of the medical appointment was "to figure out why I'm so short." Given her motivation to identify a cause and treatment for her short stature, she was quite cooperative and compliant both during a physical examination, as well as when asked to play independently, during which time she engaged the front desk staff in playing games and also eagerly demonstrated hip hop dance moves.

Sam's physical examination revealed several characteristics consistent with her 45,X/47,XY + 21 chromosomal makeup, including short stature, depressed nasal bridge/flat face, broad neck, stocky build, low set hairline, and brachycephaly (i.e., flattened back of the skull or head), but per parental report, other than resolved speech delay, she had normal cognitive development and intellect. Genital exam revealed completely typical female Tanner 1 external genitalia with normal urethral meatus and hymen and no palpable hernia or gonads. The abdominal and pelvic ultrasound showed normal kidneys and a prepubertal uterus, with only one gonad visualized. The gonad was small, 0.2 cc by 1.3 cm in greatest dimension, with no masses or follicles.

Sam's parents were seen independently from Sam to discuss her complicated diagnosis. The chromosome result report was reviewed by our genetic counselor, and it was explained that typically individuals have 46 chromosomes in all cells of their body. However, the results for Sam showed two different cell lines, which is known as "mosaicism." That is, in some of Sam's cells, there is a missing X or Y chromosome (i.e., 45,X) and in other cells there is an extra chromosome (i.e., 47,XY,+21 or trisomy 21). Sam's mosaic sex chromosome complement (i.e., X/XY) can result in a spectrum of phenotypic findings from classical Turner syndrome features with typical female genitalia to mixed gonadal dysgenesis (MGD; a diagnosis in which a chromosomal abnormality causes a child to be born with two different gonads, often a testicle and an underdeveloped "streak" gonad) with various levels of atypical genital development. Because Sam had no evidence of virilization (i.e., masculinized features such as an enlarged clitoris) on examination, and her pelvic ultrasound revealed some Müllerian structures (i.e., female internal reproductive tract), her diagnosis is most consistent with Turner syndrome with Y chromosome mosaicism. Initial discussion was about the typical findings in Turner syndrome and need for other screening.

We then moved on to the complicated additional issues regarding gonadectomy (i.e., removal of gonads). Specifically, we discussed the traditional recommendation for gonadectomy in the setting of Y chromosome material due to concern for tumor (i.e., gonadoblastoma) risk. We also highlighted controversies surrounding gonadectomy, which include concerns about removing potentially functional gonadal tissue from patients who are too young to participate in decision-making about surgery. We discussed alternatives to gonadectomy, namely, ultrasound observation, but acknowledged that ultrasound has not been fully evaluated as a tumor screening modality in this situation [17]. Last, our team discussed the theoretical potential for spontaneous puberty and fertility.

Given the presence of trisomy 21, Sam's parents asked specific questions regarding whether Sam had Down syndrome. Our genetic counselor explained that Sam's chromosome makeup would be described as mosaic Down-Turner syndrome, but that an actual clinical diagnosis of Turner syndrome or Down syndrome would depend on the phenotypic features observed. Even though we know that Sam's blood cells have two different patterns of chromosomes, we cannot determine which type of cell makes up each system of Sam's body. Because Sam's intellectual development is on target, she does not have the "expected" Down syndrome developmental delays. We reviewed reports in the literature of individuals with similar karyotypes that have been noted to have intelligence in the normal range, but did discuss the possibility that Sam may be at a higher risk for learning problems in the future.

Management

Throughout the course of this first multidisciplinary sex development clinic visit, parents were intermittently tearful, expressing fear that the rarity of Sam's diagnosis meant that there was little guidance regarding clinical management and expectant outcomes. Parents also reported that Sam's gender-nonconforming behaviors remained consistent across different contexts and persistent over time, and they had noticed increased verbal insistence of "wanting to be a boy." Parents reasoned that the presence of Y chromosome material may account for gender nonconformity, stating "well, I guess it all makes sense now why she's always been more like a boy." Recommendations provided at this initial multidisciplinary appointment included initiating growth hormone treatment given Sam's ongoing distress related to her short stature, as well as being seen within Turner Clinic for full cardiology, audiology, and ophthalmology evaluations. Additional laboratory tests were also ordered, including anti-Müllerian hormone (AMH), luteinizing hormone (LH), follicle-stimulating hormone (FSH), estradiol, testosterone, lipids, and complete metabolic panel, to complete the initial screening needed for Turner syndrome diagnosis (thyroid function studies and celiac screening had been performed recently during short stature evaluation) and to evaluate gonadal function, to help guide recommendations for potential gonadectomy and fertility potential. Sam was also referred for a gastroenterology evaluation in the context of a recent positive celiac screen and strong family history. Given the trisomy 21 cell line, possible future referral to hematology/oncology also was considered. In addition, parents expressed interest in bringing Sam in for a full psychological evaluation in the context of her increased insistence in asserting a male gender identity and parents considering whether social gender transition may be indicated.

Over the course of the next 4 months, Sam was evaluated in the multidisciplinary Turner Clinic, by gastroenterology, and parents returned to the multidisciplinary sex development clinic for a more thorough discussion about managing gonadal tissue.

In addition, Sam, her parents, and her sister were seen for a total of five sessions by our psychologist for a comprehensive psychological evaluation. As part of the evaluation, parents were seen for one session alone to discuss their emergent concerns for GD. They reported that Sam had already noticed growth since starting growth hormone treatment and was very happy and excited to see changes in height. However, one night as Sam was preparing for bed, she looked sullen and sad and when questioned by parents, shared, "I'm still sad because I really want to be a boy." Parents validated Sam's feelings, sharing with her that "there are options if that's what you really want." Once parents opened the door to discuss Sam's desires, she immediately shared, "I want to change my name. I want to tell everyone at school, and I want to use the boys' bathroom." Sam did express understanding when parents informed her that she would be meeting with the psychologist from the clinic who could help their family make a plan.

Parents specifically sought guidance on considerations for preparing for a social gender transition. Discussions centered on safety and degree of support within Sam's school and community. Sam's father was the assistant head of the private school she attended and, from his experience, felt that school administration would be supportive of Sam transitioning to a male gender role. It was recommended that parents connect with the GSDP program manager who is active in providing onsite professional development for school administration, teachers, and staff around issues of gender diversity, and also could help connect Sam's parents with other families who have supported their children in pursuing social gender transition. It was discussed that there is no "right way" to approach planning for a social gender transition and much of the decision-making process would be informed by Sam's desires and preferred timeline for transition, as well as Sam and her family's comfort level and readiness to respond to possible adversity taking into consideration the level of support from Sam's school and community. Evaluation with Sam would elucidate her understanding of gender development, including gender identity and expression, desires for transition, and preparedness to respond to possible social adversity.

Having already met our psychologist in the multidisciplinary sex development clinic and been informed by parents that she would be helping the family plan for social gender transition, Sam was immediately at ease and eager to discuss desires for transition during each of the sessions attended, accompanied by mother. Sam's mother shared that Sam "was just so happy to know we're making a plan." Over the course of the evaluation, Sam consistently maintained a positive, friendly, and engaging demeanor and presented in a stereotypically masculine fashion with regard to grooming, attire, and mannerisms. Cognitive and social developments were appropriate for age.

Upon interview, Sam expressed a desire to use "he/him/his" versus "she/her/hers" pronouns during evaluation—mother was in agreement with masculine pronoun use and reported that immediate family members had started to use masculine pronouns at home. Sam jumped in to share excitedly, "they're doing a pretty good job!" Sam also stated that he wanted to change his name, but had yet to decide from an extensive list of possibilities. Thus, he agreed to continue using Sam but requested check-ins at the start of subsequent sessions "in case I've picked a new name." Sam's mother raised his sister's concern that using a preferred name would be difficult to remember and asked Sam why he wanted to change his name when "Sam" is often considered a "boys' name." Sam was clear in communicating that even though "Sam" is a boys' name, to him, it is a reminder of the name given to him "when I was a girl."

Mother shared that Sam presented to Turner Clinic with the following stated purpose: "I'm here to get taller and because I want to be a boy." And in the context of psychoeducation about his Turner syndrome diagnosis and learning that he likely would not go through a spontaneous puberty and would need exogenous estrogen to initiate female puberty, Sam had asked whether he could "take boy medicines sometime in my teens" instead and "become a boy." Sam expressed a strong desire to develop male secondary sexual characteristics and was curious about whether male hormones would lead to his "growing a penis," which he expressly desired.

Diagnostically, Sam met full *DSM-5* criteria for Gender Dysphoria in Children with a co-occurring DSD condition. No other behavioral or emotional concerns were endorsed by Sam, his parents, or Sam's classroom teacher. Given that parents and Sam were all committed to moving forward with a social gender transition, it was recommended that the family have regular follow-up to support them in planning and implementing the transition. Of note, by the time psychological evaluation was completed, parents already had met with Sam's classroom teacher and school administrators who all were in full support of social gender transition. Parents also decided to allow Sam to dictate when and how he would like to disclose plans for transition to classmates. In their preliminary discussions with Sam, he expressed desire to transition before the current school year ended. His current plan was to ask his teacher to read the book "Be Who You Are" [18], which is about a birth-assigned male child who transitions to living as female, after which he will explain that he "feels how the character in the book feels, just opposite… born a girl but really feel like a boy."

Brief Literature Review

Classical Turner syndrome is classified as a sex chromosome DSD and affects approximately 1 in 2500 females [19]. It is a genetic condition characterized by X-chromosome monosomy (i.e., 45,X), short stature, and complete gonadal dysgenesis, usually leading to ovarian failure, lack of spontaneous pubertal development, and infertility. A variable number of other clinical features may be present, including webbed neck, cardiovascular defects, kidney anomalies, hearing loss, propensity to develop autoimmune diseases, and selective cognitive impairment. External genitalia are typical of a female, and female gender identity has been exclusively reported in the literature [17]. Approximately 50% (and suspected to be higher) of all women with Turner syndrome have some type of mosaicism (e.g., 45,X/46,XX), and approximately 6% have mosaic 45,X/46,XY with as high as 12%

having some Y chromosome material present [20, 21]. Mosaicism is typically a sporadic chromosome change, and there are no known factors that could cause or increase risk for mosaicism.

In girls with Turner syndrome and Y chromosome mosaicism (i.e., 45,X/46,XY karyotype), there is an increased risk for germ cell cancer, typically prompting recommendation for gonadectomy to prevent this progression [22]. There are no published reports documenting GD in girls with Turner syndrome with Y chromosome mosaicism; however, the clinical practice guidelines for the care of girls and women with Turner syndrome state, "the patient and/or her parents should be informed of the finding of Y chromosome material with the utmost sensitivity regarding gender identity issues to minimize psychological harm" [17]. No other mention of gender identity or GD in this population is referenced.

It is important to note that the 45,X/46,XY karyotype can be seen in a wide spectrum of phenotypes. This includes female-typical genitalia as in Turner syndrome, incomplete virilization of external genitalia due to mixed gonadal dysgenesis (MGD), or typical male genitalia, which actually is the most common phenotype. In the MGD population, genital ambiguity at birth often necessitates genetic and endocrine evaluation and a deliberate decision-making process for sex assignment, taking into account the degree of virilization, surgical options, gonadal functioning/need for lifelong hormone replacement therapy, potential for fertility, and views of the family regarding gender of rearing. GD in this cohort is common, with variable reported rates of 12% [23], 29% [24], and 55% [25]. In the reports by Szarras-Czapnik et al. [23] and Reiner [25], those raised male had a male gender identity whereas GD emerged among those raised female. Since the same 45,X/46,XY karyotype encompasses a broad range of phenotypes, it is important to consider this continuum in evaluation and management of a patient with this karyotype.

As previously highlighted, mosaicism in Turner syndrome is common. However, mosaicism for trisomy 21 is less common with an estimated prevalence of 2–4% mosaicism [26]. Double aneuploidy, the occurrence of two numerical chromosome abnormalities, such as that of 45,X and 47,XX/XY+21 is rare. Approximately 50 cases have been reported in the literature [27, 28]. Clinical phenotype was variable ranging from phenotypically typical male to Down syndrome to Down-Turner syndrome. Of interest, the majority of cases were described to have features most consistent with Down syndrome, and no reported cases described phenotypes as solely Turner syndrome or normal female phenotype (as was the case for Sam). Of 44 cases with a documented karyotype, 9 cases had identified Y material. All of these cases were reported as having either male (7/9), or ambiguous (2/9), genitalia [27].

Clinical Pearls/Pitfalls

In many respects, assessment and treatment of GD in Sam's case was fairly straightforward, given the lack of co-occurring psychiatric conditions and in the context of a supportive, affirming family and school environment. Sam presented with a persistent history of gender nonconformity that remained consistent and stable over time, with body dysphoria emerging as he developed deeper understanding of differences between male and female bodies. Sam's parents were accepting of his gender-nonconforming behaviors and supported his choosing to express gender how he felt most comfortable in terms of clothing and hairstyle, even as a young child. They were not particularly concerned with identifying a reason why Sam was gender-nonconforming; rather, parents' primary concern was whether they were doing everything they could to support Sam to promote positive health outcomes. In addition, parents were savvy consumers of healthcare and sought out psychological consultation early and, thus, were well informed of both social and medical transition options available to Sam to alleviate GD, if and when they became indicated. Parents also appropriately followed Sam's lead in dictating both need for additional psychological consultation and evaluation, as well as deciding on optimal timing for social gender transition.

Moving forward, Sam and his family appear well positioned and prepared for social gender transition. Making decisions regarding medical management of Sam's unique condition will be more difficult. Specifically, Sam's parents were seen again in the sex development clinic after additional laboratory tests were obtained. The most predictive laboratory for gonadal function at Sam's age point (i.e., anti-Müllerian hormone) was unfavorable for spontaneous puberty. Thus, considerations for surgical removal versus expectant management of the gonads in the setting of Y chromosome material were discussed in the context of Sam's longstanding history of gender nonconformity and GD. Given the risk of gonadoblastoma and low likelihood of spontaneous female puberty (which, currently, would be highly undesired by and distressing for Sam) and fertility, we shared the impression that there is likely more risk than benefit to expectant management. Should Sam's parents elect to proceed with irreversible gonadectomy, they also will need to decide whether to cryopreserve Sam's gonadal tissue via experimental protocol for future advanced fertility options.

As the team providing multidisciplinary care to Sam and his family, we were challenged to reflect on whether there would have been any utility to recommending genetic and endocrine work-up to parents at the time of initial psychological consultation given parental report that Sam was "small for her age," and short stature being associated with Turner syndrome, a sex chromosome DSD. Had work-up been recommended, discovery of Sam's 45,X/47,XY + 21 karyotype potentially could have occurred 6 months prior to when it actually was discovered, time that may be significant in cases where gonadoblastoma is present. However, GD has not been reported in the literature as associated with classical Turner syndrome, nor have there been reports of GD among Turner syndrome with Y chromosome mosaicism. Thus, the impact of Sam's karyotype on gender nonconformity and GD remains unclear.

While GD may be observed among youth with DSD conditions at a higher rate compared to the general population, there is little understanding of the true etiology of gender identity development and GD. As 45,X/47,XY,+21 karyotype is rare, there are no reports of GD among patients with similar karyotypes. However, as previously stated, GD has been described in association with 45,X/46,XY MGD [23–25, 29]; thus, although the mechanism is unknown, it is possible that the

47,XY,+21 cell line, or a possible undiscovered 46,XY cell line, may have had some effect on the developing brain and other tissue which may be impacting Sam's gender identification. Regardless of whether there is an identifiable biological "explanation" for GD or not, recommendations for gender-affirming care do not change. However, we recognize that having a biological explanation for gender nonconformity or GD may be helpful to some parents who, unlike Sam's parents, may struggle to accept their child's gender-nonconforming behaviors.

Perhaps the most important message with regard to clinical practice illustrated by Sam's case is the immense benefit of having joint multidisciplinary gender-DSD programs with the same specialists providing care for both patient populations in cases where there is comorbidity between GD and DSD conditions. In Sam's case, his parents were able to lean on our team psychologist for support as they initially learned about Sam's atypical karyotype given their existing therapeutic relationship. Additionally, Sam's DSD condition typically prompts recommendation for gonadectomy, and how parents elect to proceed with management of gonadal tissue will impact medical treatment for GD, in the event that Sam's GD persists into adolescence and he desires physical transition with hormones. Having all members of the multidisciplinary GSDP team well versed in considerations related to management of both GD and DSD was invaluable in providing care to Sam and his family.

Key Learning Points

1. Unless there is a physical indication for genetic or endocrine evaluation of sex chromosomes and androgen exposure, youth presenting with primary concerns for GD are not currently recommended to undergo medical work-up.
2. In cases of GD in the context of a co-occurring DSD condition, involving a multidisciplinary team is important for continuity of care.
3. Whether or not GD co-occurs with a DSD condition does not change the clinical approach to affirm a child's gender identity and support them to live as they feel most comfortable.
4. Social gender transition among prepubertal youth remains controversial, and considering a multitude of factors, including a child's emotional, social, and psychological functioning, degree of family and community support, and preparedness to cope with potential adversity, is important when helping families make decisions about the benefits of a social gender transition.

References

1. Lee PA, Houk CP, Ahmed SF, Hughes IA. International consensus conference on intersex organized by the Lawson Wilkins Pediatric Endocrine Society and the European Society for Paediatric Endocrinology. Consensus statement on management of intersex disorders. International Consensus Conference on Intersex. Pediatrics. 2006;118(2):e488–500.
2. American Psychiatric Association. Diagnostic and statistical manual of mental disorders. 5th ed. Arlington, VA: American Psychiatric Association; 2013.

3. Meyer-Bahlburg HF. Sex steroids and variants of gender identity. Endocrinol Metab Clin N Am. 2013;42(3):435–52.
4. Chen D, Hidalgo MA, Leibowitz S, Leininger J, Simons L, Finlayson C, et al. Multidisciplinary care for gender-diverse youth: a narrative review and unique model of gender-affirming care. Transgender Health. July 2016;1(1):117–23.
5. Hsieh S, Leininger J. Resource list: clinical care programs for gender-nonconforming children and adolescents. Pediatr Ann. 2014;43(6):238–44.
6. Drescher J, Byne W. Gender dysphoric/gender variant (GD/GV) children and adolescents: summarizing what we know and what we have yet to learn. J Homosex. 2012;59(3):501–10.
7. Steensma TD, Biemond R, de Boer F, Cohen-Kettenis PT. Desisting and persisting gender dysphoria after childhood: a qualitative follow-up study. Clin Child Psychol Psychiatry. 2011;16(4):499–516.
8. Steensma TD, McGuire JK, Kreukels BP, Beekman AJ, Cohen-Kettenis PT. Factors associated with desistence and persistence of childhood gender dysphoria: a quantitative follow-up study. J Am Acad Child Adolesc Psychiatry. 2013;52(6):582–90.
9. Zucker KJ, Wood H, Singh D, Bradley SJ. A developmental, biopsychosocial model for the treatment of children with gender identity disorder. J Homosex. 2012;59(3):369–97.
10. Hidalgo MA, Ehrensaft D, Tishelman AC, Clark LF, Garofalo R, Rosenthal SM, et al. The gender affirmative model: what we know and what we aim to learn. Hum Dev. 2013;56(5):285–90.
11. de Vries AL, Cohen-Kettenis PT. Clinical management of gender dysphoria in children and adolescents: the Dutch approach. J Homosex. 2012;59(3):301–20.
12. Edwards-Leeper L, Leibowitz S, Sangganjanavanich VF. Affirmative practice with transgender and gender nonconforming youth: expanding the model. Psychol Sex Orientat Gender Diversity. 2016;3(2):165–72.
13. Ryan C, Russell ST, Huebner D, Diaz R, Sanchez J. Family acceptance in adolescence and the health of LGBT young adults. J Child Adolesc Psychiatr Nurs. 2010;23(4):205–13.
14. Olson KR, Durwood L, DeMeules M, McLaughlin KA. Health of transgender children who are supported in their identities. Pediatrics. 2016;137(3):e20153223.
15. Ehrensaft D. Gender born, gender made. New York: The Experiment; 2011.
16. Brill S, Pepper R. The transgender child. San Francisco, CA: Cleis Press; 2008.
17. Bondy CA. Care of girls and women with turner syndrome: a guideline of the turner syndrome study group. J Clin Endocrinol Metab. 2007;92(1):10–25.
18. Carr J. Be who you are! AuthorHouse: Bloomington, IN; 2010.
19. Hall JG, Gilchrist DM. Turner syndrome and its variants. Pediatr Clin N Am. 1990;37(6):1421–40.
20. Freriks K, Timmers HJ, Netea-Maier RT, Beerendonk CC, Otten BJ, van Alfen-van der Velden JA, et al. Buccal cell FISH and blood PCR-Y detect high rates of X chromosomal mosaicism and Y chromosomal derivatives in patients with turner syndrome. Eur J Med Genet. 2013;56(9):497–501.
21. Ackermann A, Bamba V. Current controversies in turner syndrome: genetic testing, assisted reproduction, and cardiovascular risks. J Clin Transl Endocrinol. 2014;1(3):61–5.
22. van der Zwan YG, Biermann K, Wolffenbuttel KP, Cools M, Looijenga LH. Gonadal maldevelopment as risk factor for germ cell cancer: towards a clinical decision model. Eur Urol. 2015;67(4):692–701.
23. Szarras-Czapnik M, Lew-Starowicz Z, Zucker KJ. A psychosexual follow-up study of patients with mixed or partial gonadal dysgenesis. J Pediatr Adolesc Gynecol. 2007;20(6):333–8.
24. Furtado PS, Moraes F, Lago R, Barros LO, Toralles MB, Barroso U Jr. Gender dysphoria associated with disorders of sex development. Nat Rev Urol. 2012;9(11):620–7.
25. Reiner WG. Gender identity and sex-of-rearing in children with disorders of sexual differentiation. J Pediatr Endocrinol Metab. 2005;18(6):549–53.
26. Devlin L, Morrison PJ. Mosaic down’s syndrome prevalence in a complete population study. Arch Dis Child. 2004;89(12):1177–8.

27. Ryu SW, Lee G, Baik CS, Shim SH, Kim JT, Lee JS, et al. Down-turner syndrome (45,X/47,XY,+21): case report and review. Korean J Lab Med. 2010;30(2):195–200.
28. Van Buggenhout GJ, Hamel BC, Trommelen JC, Mieloo H, Smeets DF. Down-turner syndrome: case report and review. J Med Genet. 1994;31(10):807–10.
29. Ocal G, Berberoğlu M, Siklar Z, Bilir P. Gender dysphoria and gender change in an adolescent with 45,X/46,XY mixed gonadal dysgenesis. Exp Clin Endocrinol Diabetes. 2009;117(6):301–4.

Chapter 7
Prepubertal Children with Gender Dysphoria: A Case to Illustrate the Management of Co-occurring Attention Deficit Hyperactivity Disorder and Disruptive Behavior Disorders

David Call

Introduction

Children who are prepubertal *are* increasingly presenting in clinical practice having already transitioned socially to a gender different from what was assigned to them at birth [1]. The concept of how to best assist families of prepubertal children with decision-making around social gender transition is still debated among professionals in the field, as there is no formal empirically supported, evidence-based intervention that definitively leads to positive emotional, social, and psychological development for the long term.

As noted in an earlier chapter (Chap. 2) in this casebook, there are ethical debates surrounding gender transition for children. To summarize, proponents of supporting a social gender transition in childhood have described the benefits of helping a child live authentically from an earlier age, and there is research to support that at that moment in time, anxiety and depressive symptomatology of these socially transitioned children is equal to that of siblings and non-GD control groups [2]. However, opponents have indicated that a social gender transition in these children may be premature, considering the only prospective evidence in the literature suggests that children presenting with gender identity concerns are more likely to not demonstrate gender dysphoria later on once puberty is experienced [3]. The latter argument suggests that a premature social transition itself may influence the child in a direction that might actually not be authentic later on and perhaps shuttles children onto a path of medical and surgical intervention.

Approaching each child individually with a balanced, yet affirming, assessment that appreciates the nuance of each family situation has also been described [4].

D. Call, MD
Division of Psychiatry and Behavioral Sciences, Children's National Health System, Washington, DC, USA
e-mail: dcall@childrensnational.org

A. Janssen, S. Leibowitz (eds.), *Affirmative Mental Health Care for Transgender and Gender Diverse Youth*, https://doi.org/10.1007/978-3-319-78307-9_7

Indeed, understanding the potential co-occurring psychiatric and potential psychiatric issues that exist for a given child would *seem* important when assisting families with social gender transition for children at this age. This chapter focuses on ADHD as a co-occurring psychiatric condition and the clinical implications associated with it to guide assessment and clinical decision-making.

Summary of Key Clinical Questions

1. To what extent can the clinician parse out the diagnostic complexities when assessing a child with gender identity concerns presenting with ADHD symptomatology?
2. For prepubertal children with co-occurring ADHD and GD, what are the potential implications that the provider and parent must take into account when considering a social gender transition for that child?
3. How does the combination of ADHD and gender dysphoria impact a child's social development or sense of self?

Co-occurring Attention Deficit Hyperactivity Disorder and/or Disruptive Behavior Disorders in Prepubertal Gender Dysphoric Children

Early studies indicated that children with gender dysphoria have increased rates of behavioral issues, but the cause of these issues can be multifactorial and not necessarily as a result of having a comorbid diagnosis of ADHD [5]. Wallien et al. found in a sample of 120 children aged 4–11 years old that 23% met criteria for a single psychiatric diagnosis and 29% met criteria for multiple diagnoses. More specifically, the study found that 23% of those children that met criteria for GID also met criteria for a disruptive disorder (ADHD, oppositional defiant disorder, conduct disorder) [6]. In older children, De Vries et al. looked to examine psychiatric comorbidities in a group of 105 adolescents (12–17 years old) with either a diagnosis of GID or having subthreshold symptoms for the full diagnosis of GID and found 11.4% to have a diagnosis of any disruptive behavior disorder (ADHD and/or oppositional defiant disorder) [7]. A recent chart review study looked at rates of gender variance as indicated by parents completing the Child Behavior Checklist, which asks if their child sometimes or often "wishes to be the opposite sex," and found higher rates of gender variance in a group of children with diagnosis of ADHD or 6.64 times as likely when compared to a typically developing control group [8].

Of note, recent studies have indicated that children with GD are more likely to demonstrate co-occurring diagnoses with internalizing symptoms (e.g., anxiety and depression) versus externalizing (e.g., behavioral acting out, impulsivity), the latter of which are what attention deficit hyperactivity disorder (ADHD) manifests mostly as [5, 9]. However, the literature indicates that peer relations for clinically referred children with GD are poorer than for non-referred children [5, 9]. The quality of peer relationships was the strongest predictor for emotional and behavior problems in Canadian children in a cross-national study looking at children with GD in Canada and the Netherlands [9]. Understanding the child's behavioral symptoms and considering whether they are derived from the distress that comes from gender dysphoria versus being part of a comorbid psychiatric condition can be challenging for children presenting with both. Many symptoms of ADHD and disruptive behaviors may also be seen in a variety of presentations outside of those formally diagnosed with ADHD or a disruptive behavior disorder. One could question inattention as a manifestation of ADHD, distress, or anxiety of being discovered and/or bullied as another gender or a combination of both. It is not unusual for parents to initially want to encourage a child to conform to gender norms and stereotypes, and one may wonder if this behavior is more related to the distress of having to express themselves in a way that does not fit their gender identity than being consistent with a disruptive behavior disorder.

ADHD can have implications on children's social functioning, as some evidence suggests that children with ADHD are more likely to be rejected by their peer group [10]. Evidence also suggests that children with ADHD may have additional difficulties in peer relationships or be less socially preferred by their peers [11]. For cisgender children with ADHD, impaired social decision-making has been found to mediate the association between ADHD and social development [12]. For children with gender dysphoria and ADHD, it may be less likely for the child to inhibit their impulses to express their gender identity, whereas other non-ADHD children may be more likely to hide their gender identity as they learn about societal or cultural pressures to conform or hide their gender identity [8]. This may also have implications in some of the decisions that families and children may make in regard to how they express their gender, to whom they disclose their identities to, and may have implications on their decisions to socially transition. Therefore, with the added stigma or internal struggles that GD children face, it seems prudent to take this into account when children present with both ADHD and GD in clinical practice.

Social gender transition in this age group can come with decisions regarding whether or not the child is "stealth" (living in the gender role they affirm at the time without others knowing), and many parents opt to protect their children by moving to a new school or community where the child is not known to have previously been a different gender. Parents also question who or when to tell and how to accept their child's gender diversity without inadvertently reinforcing shame by sending the message that the transition is a secret. Therefore, higher-order social decision-making constructs are often necessary when guiding families with these complex decisions.

Case Report

Diagnosis and Assessment

At the initial point of assessment, Dana presented as a 6-year-old birth-assigned male who identified as female and referred to herself with female (she/her) pronouns. She presented for an initial evaluation with her parents over concerns that she had worsening self-esteem and was very sensitive to how the slightest action might result in other kids making fun of her. Her parents were also concerned about Dana's behaviors and described her as being very energetic and impulsive and having difficulty maintaining much focus in activities. They were concerned about a possible diagnosis of ADHD and how this was playing a role in her social difficulties. Dana was initially diagnosed with gender dysphoria at the age of 4, presenting with a history of significant and consistent gender nonconforming behaviors and interests. Dana previously lived in another state, where she was frequently teased and bullied by peers and adults in the community. Since relocating to a new area, Dana's parents talked with her about not disclosing her identity as being transgender; however, Dana has on a number of occasions impulsively revealed her identity as "transgender" and received both positive and negative responses from peers. In this case, Dana experienced potential rejection not only from revealing her gender identity as being transgender but also potentially from the difficulties that ADHD created in forming and maintaining peer relationships.

In school, social activities, and family events and with friends, Dana presented as a girl, had changed her name from Daniel, and used female pronouns instead of male pronouns. Dana's family recently relocated for work purposes and had been living in the region over the past year. During that time, Dana's parents had been concerned that she had decreased self-esteem as evidenced by becoming much more self-conscious about her looks and appearance. Much of this concern appeared to center around Dana being able to present as more feminine and be perceived by others as a girl. This was in the context of Dana recently disclosing to other peers in the neighborhood that she identifies as a *transgender girl*, stating "I told them I have a girl brain in a boy's body." Although some of her friends responded positively and with support, one peer told his parents and others that Dana is not a "real girl." Her parents also noted that after this disclosure, Dana became more isolative and less interested in being social with peers. They did not notice any changes in sleep patterns or appetite. There was no history of self-injurious behavior or suicidal ideation.

In addition, parents were concerned about Dana's behavioral issues and were told by other providers that she might also have ADHD. In terms of inattentive symptoms, Dana's parents described her having difficulty paying close attention during tasks related to school and rushing through work. They noticed that she had much difficulty sustaining attention in not only school tasks but even in play, giving an example of how she could not even watch a short 20- to 25-min cartoon show in its entirety because of how easily distracted she gets. They described her as being quite disorganized and often resisting activities she knew would take a significant amount of time or effort. She very frequently lost or misplaced toys and supplies for school. It was not unusual for her parents to have to remind her repeatedly to do a task or chore that they asked her to do.

In terms of hyperactivity and impulsivity symptoms, her parents noted that she was very fidgety and had much difficulty sitting still in school or when out in public. They noted in play that she tended to be louder and more active than the other kids and would have difficulty slowing down when asked to walk or when the group needed to be quiet. Her parents noted that she often talked excessively and would interrupt conversations. They also noticed sometimes it caused difficulty when playing with groups of kids as she would have problems with waiting her turn. Dana's parents noted that these have been concerns that have been chronic and predated the family's move and her social gender transition. They also noted that these problem areas occurred both in school, at home, and during extracurricular activities but also improved somewhat when she had more individual attention from adults.

In terms of oppositional behaviors, her parents noted that at times she would frequently actively defy rules or request by adults, particularly if she was in the midst of a play activity that she enjoyed. They also noted that it would seem as if Dana would frequently deliberately do things to annoy others. However, they did not note that Dana ever seemed overly angry, resentful, spiteful, or vindictive. They also noted that she did not argue with adults over what one might expect from a child her age. Since socially transitioning to living as female, and allowing Dana to express her gender in the way she asserted (such as through clothes and hairstyle), they noted an improvement in her temper tantrums in public situations compared previously, when they report limiting her gender expression.

Psychiatric History

Dana did have an early history of speech delay, as she did not start using single words until she was approximately 2½ years of age. Her parents noted that Dana seemed to have much more difficulty with expressive language but seemed to understand what others were saying very well. Dana was also toilet trained around that time and exhibited bowel control for a few months but then started to refuse to use the toilet. She was assessed by occupational therapy at that time and was given a diagnosis of sensory processing disorder. Through speech and occupational therapy, Dana started to speak more expressively and regained bowel control by 3.5 years of age. Previous providers were concerned about a possible diagnosis of autism spectrum disorder given the speech delay and some of the sensory issues observed, but it was determined that she did not meet the criteria for autism spectrum disorder after psychological evaluation. However, during that evaluation it was determined that Dana had a diagnosis of gender dysphoria and a possible diagnosis of attention deficit hyperactivity disorder. Dana had never been on psychotropic medications, as the impairment in functioning at that time was not believed to be severe enough to warrant pharmacologic intervention and Dana was referred for individual therapy with the goals of further exploring her gender identity, ways to express her gender identity, and managing some of the difficulties that arose when she experienced negative reactions from others in regard to her transition.

During the initial psychiatric interview with Dana, she was initially quite shy, and we started the interview by discussing some of her general interests. Dana was very interested in talking about her interests in various video games and dolls. In particular, Dana had described interests in a popular brand of dolls which feature characters that wear different fashion designs. Dana talked about the fact that she had started making doll clothes with her mother's help and hoped to be a designer someday. Other interests of Dana's included being outside with her friends in the neighborhood playing games such as "tag" and "hide and seek." In particular, Dana described one of her neighborhood friends as her "best friend" and states they often played at each other's houses. Dana's parents revealed that this friend and her family were aware of her assigned sex at birth being male, yet her living as female, and have been very supportive.

When asked further about her interests, Dana states that she "always" liked playing with "girl toys" but went on to state that there were "lots of mean people" in where she previously lived. She stated that people were not as mean in where she lived presently but did state she got very upset when her friend told her she "wasn't really a girl," after disclosing to him that she is "transgender." More recently, Dana described often playing by herself because, "I don't like the games everyone else plays." When asked what games she plays by herself, she stated that she "plays catch" and she did not like playing some of the sports that the other kids engage in. In regard to some of the behavioral concerns her parents raised, she stated, "sometimes I don't clean my room and I play with my toys instead and get in trouble."

Dana's parents described further concerns about her behaviors both chronically and more recently. They feel like Dana may be "embarrassed" about being transgender and is now more concerned about "being able to pass as a girl." They noted that previously, Dana would often be more outgoing and want to be the center of attention but more recently had been "getting more quiet." Over the previous month, they felt that there have been some more positive changes, where they saw Dana appear as more "happy" and wanting to play with toys again. Previously, right after the move, she seemed more indifferent. They stated that they had seen her have more energy and be "more full of life," as she has settled into her new home. However, the parents were worried about how things would progress in the future. Although Dana had not seemed to talk about her gender identity with others much since the incident with the peer, they wondered if she felt some shame about being "transgender." They also worried how she would handle future situations when someone questions her gender identity.

In terms of medical history, there were no current or past concerns. They reported a family history on the paternal side of depression, but no known family history of ADHD or other psychiatric conditions.

Gender Development History

In terms of Dana's gender development, her parents noted that from a very early age, Dana had always expressed an interest in toys that were more stereotypically viewed as being girl's toys, such as princess and female character dolls. Her parents noted that she would get very excited about watching shows and movies that featured more feminine characters, such as princesses. By the age of 4, Dana was asking to wear dresses and would cry when shopping with her mother and getting clothes from the boys' section instead of the girls'. Given how upset she would get, they initially allowed Dana to wear some girls' outfits at home, but not in public. Initially, given some of the sensory issues that were identified between the ages of 2 and 3 years of age, her parents believed that her interest in girls' clothing has more to do with a tactile sensitivity. Around this time, after Dana had an evaluation and was given the diagnosis of gender dysphoria, they allowed her to wear girls' outfits in public and stopped trying to get her to wear clothes from the boys' section. Her parents noted that this seemed to improve her behavioral outbursts, and Dana further wanted to explore other ways of presenting herself, such as painting her nails and wanting to style her hair in longer and more stereotypical feminine styles. Her parents also noted that around the age of 4, they first recall hearing Dana make statements regarding how she identified herself, stating "I am a girl!" and, more recently, they stated that she typically made statements like this on a daily basis. In pretend play, they observed Dana imitating female characters and had never seen her imitating male characters. Furthermore, in terms of social relationships, her closest friends have been girls, and she has been active in an after-school club for girls.

When Dana was first diagnosed with gender dysphoria, her parents allowed her to socially transition to living as a female by wearing the clothes she wanted to wear and to go by her chosen name, changing from the more masculine "Daniel," and telling family and friends that she is a girl. This led to some difficulties, as some members of her local community did not agree with her expressing her gender as a girl. Dana herself recalled other peers "saying mean things to me" and also identified that she felt sad "because people didn't believe me." Her parents noted that not only was she victim to teasing by peers, but many of the adults in the community would ignore her or prevent her from playing with their children. When Dana's family moved, they made a decision that they would not tell many people in their new community that Dana is transgender but that she is simply a girl. However, Dana started to tell her classmates at school that she is "transgender," and this led to some peers not understanding the meaning of that and telling her that she isn't really a girl. This had led more recently to Dana becoming much more focused on wanting to make sure she looks like a girl and feeling more concerned about others finding out that she was born a boy.

Psychosocial Factors

At the time of presentation, Dana lived in a single-family home with her mother and father. She is an only child and her parents had her as a planned pregnancy when both were in their early 20s. Dana is Caucasian, and her family did not have any specific religious beliefs. In terms of schooling, Dana was in kindergarten at a public school. She enjoyed art class the most. She enjoyed designing new clothes with her mother's help for her dolls. Academically, Dana did have some struggles with completing assignments and maintaining a focus on classroom activities, although they were not entirely demanding given that it was kindergarten level. Her work was often described as being rushed and messy, and she was often redirected for talking out of turn, staying in her seat, and following classroom rules. She was receiving occupational therapy and speech therapy and was making academic progress despite some of these issues.

Mental Status Exam

During the initial evaluation, Dana presented wearing a more stereotypical girl's outfit (wearing a shirt with a feminine looking cartoon cat character on it, pink jacket, pink sneakers with glitter). Her hair was long and styled in a ponytail. Initially, she appeared shy and stayed close to her mother, hiding her face at first when the interviewers from the team introduced themselves. However, Dana warmed up quickly and became more engaged with interviewers providing appropriate eye contact and answering questions appropriately. She was quite hyperactive in the office and had much difficulty sitting still for more than a couple of minutes at a time. Dana is cooperative and responded well to redirection but would often need to be reminded repeatedly throughout the interview to stay on task. Her speech was spontaneous, and she exhibited some articulation issues but overall was intelligible. The volume of her speech was loud at times, particularly when she was excited to talk about some of her favorite toys. During conversations, she would also interrupt the interviewer at times. When not sitting in the chair and talking about some of her interests, she would dance or twirl in excitement. Her eye contact was good throughout the conversation, and she used gestures appropriately in describing different activities that she enjoyed. Dana described her mood as being "happy" and she had an overall pleasant affect that was full in range. Her thought process was linear and concrete (developmentally appropriate), and there was no concerning thought content, such as signs of suicidal ideation, homicidal ideation, or any overt delusions noted. During the interview, she was easily distracted by different objects and toys in the office. Even when she was allowed to play with some of the toys, she has difficulty focusing on any one particular toy and shifts to a different toy every few minutes. Her diagnoses were consistent with gender dysphoria in childhood and attention deficit hyperactivity disorder, combined type.

Formulation

The formulation of Dana's presentation was as follows: Dana is a 6-year-old assigned male at birth who identifies and has socially transitioned to living as a girl who presented to the gender development program for concerns regarding inattention, hyperactivity, and self-esteem issues after a recent move to the area, a major

East Coast city. Dana's presentation was consistent with a diagnosis of gender dysphoria given her history of having a strong desire to be a girl, a consistent demonstration of distress when any stereotypical masculine items or clothing were introduced into her daily life, and an unwavering insistent expression that she *is* a girl. She had shown a number of behaviors, such as wanting to wear the clothes that are more stereotypically worn by girls, consistently imitating female characters in pretend play, and preferring toys and games that are more stereotypically favored by girls. Per Dana's parents, she had also made statements of not liking her sexual anatomy.

Dana had been subject to significant bullying and negative reactions from others, when she was living in a state that was in the middle of the country. It is notable that after allowing Dana to socially transition to living as a female, such as allowing her to wear more stereotypical girl's clothes and use a more typical feminine name, many of the behavioral issues improved. However, with her recent move to the East Coast city, Dana had also encountered some difficulty and anxiety around how she might be perceived by others. Given Dana's age, impulsivity associated with ADHD, inability to fully navigate complex social situations, and stage of development, it is not surprising that she started to tell peers about her gender identity being discrepant from her birth-assigned sex. She may not have been fully aware of the risk of having negative reactions. In addition, Dana has a number of symptoms that are consistent with a diagnosis of attention deficit hyperactivity disorder, combined type. She had also found much support in the community and from some family members that have helped give Dana a sense of acceptance. Dana's more recent symptoms of withdrawal were likely related to some of her peers' reactions to her statements and subsequently hearing a comment that peers saw her as a "half boy-half girl." This may have led her to be more self-conscious about her appearance and likely could be implicated in some of the changes in her behavior from being more extroverted to more withdrawn. More recent improvements had likely been the result of having a very supportive family that had given Dana a sense of love and acceptance.

It is not unusual in young children with anxiety to sometimes appear more active or inattentive if they are ruminating on sources of anxiety. However, parents described these symptoms as more chronic in nature and persisted despite addressing some of the concerns Dana had regarding her gender identity. At the time, Dana did not appear to meet the full criteria for a mood or anxiety disorder; however the treatment team determined that this should be closely monitored given some of the heightened awareness that Dana shows of peers and others being aware of her gender dysphoria and thus possibly encountering negative reactions as a result.

Management

After the initial evaluation, we invited the family to participate in a group program specific to families with children presenting with gender-related concerns to receive support and psychoeducation. Dana had the opportunity to participate in a playgroup that is considered to be a safe, supported space to further explore ways to express herself and socialize with other peers who may be gender nonconforming or identify as transgender like herself. At the same time, Dana's parents were able to participate in the parent support group and could meet other parents with children who are gender nonconforming or identified as transgender. This provided help for the parents on how to navigate some situations in the future that may prove difficult. For example, the group addresses how, when, and to whom Dana could disclose her gender identity status to and offered other ways for how the parents could best support their child. Since Dana's initial disclosure to some of her friends, she has not openly (per parent's knowledge) discussed her "secret" as a topic of conversation with other peers. To her parents, she continued to express concern at times about whether she looks enough like a girl and has continued to socialize in activities with her peers outside of school.

In terms of managing Dana's interests, the team supported her parent's acceptance in letting her explore her interests in play and expression. We discussed taking a child-centered approach, following Dana's lead in choices of which games to play or which clothes to wear. However, we did discuss with the parents about having appropriate boundaries and limits as they would with any child regardless of their gender identity. For example, it would be important to educate parents that it might be useful for Dana to wear appropriate shorts or undergarments underneath wearing a skirt so she does not risk exposing herself on the playground. A common theme for some of the parents was such that the children often express their gender in extreme ways, considering their hypervigilance against being perceived as the gender associated with their birth-assigned sex. Therefore, another related point of psychoeducation for the parents was to educate them on not allowing Dana to wear shoes with heels in an activity such as gym class where all kids are expected to wear sneakers.

In terms of disclosure to others about Dana's gender identity, it was recommended to get Dana's input on who she may or may not want to know about her identity. We recommended continuing to have open communication with Dana about her feelings related to how others might respond to knowing about her gender identity. Maintaining an approach that considers Dana's comfort was important, as trying to encourage Dana to hide her identity could also send a message that there is something wrong with her or lead to feelings of shame. Conversely, encouraging Dana to tell others about her identity could itself lead to increasing anxiety. Individual therapy was recommended as a way to (1) help Dana to further explore emotions around disclosure, (2) further clarify how to detect the safety of the situation when expressing her gender to those around her, and (3) provide her with an open space to reinforce the notion that she could express herself in whatever way made sense for her as she grew older (including the possibility of reverting back to living as male or even potentially adopting a nonbinary gender identity should that most authentically describe her experience in the future). Addressing the ADHD symptoms would be important in order to achieve these gender-based goals within therapy.

In terms of the concerns related to Dana's ADHD symptomatology, it was recommended that Dana receive as much structural supports in the school setting as would be appropriate for any other child with ADHD. Behavioral strategies were recommended as helpful in managing some of the concerns with inattention and impulse control. Examples included setting out structured routines for tasks such as school work and chores and the use of visual schedules that were posted to remind Dana of the tasks she needed to do during the day. These could also be used as a reference point, so that she would know what to expect later in the day. Teaching in an environment with minimal distractions was also recommended as important to help her maintain focus. Individual therapy would provide behavioral strategies to address the inattention and hyperactivity. Psychopharmacological interventions for ADHD were deferred at that point in time, but psychoeducation was provided about this intervention in the future so that the parents and treatment team could consider medication in the future depending on the presence of functional impairment associated with her ADHD.

Clinical Pearls/Pitfalls

This case illustrates a number of issues that occur when working with gender nonconforming youth in the presence of ADHD. As mentioned at the beginning of the chapter, there has only been limited data looking at the prevalence of ADHD in children with gender dysphoria. There are also limited data on the efficacy of social gender transition with children who meet criteria for GD, and therefore many complexities need to be addressed even in the absence of a co-occurring psychiatric diagnosis. Other disruptive behavioral disorders, such as oppositional defiant disorder, can also be difficult to delineate from the oppositionality that may occur with a child with gender dysphoria, who may be feeling pressure from their family, community, or society to suppress authentic interests or ways of expressing themselves in order to be more conforming with typical gender roles. When examining the core symptoms of ADHD and oppositional defiant disorder, one could potentially see an overlap between the presence of these symptoms in a child with gender dysphoria with varying different explanations for the presence of the symptoms. For example, is the child who fidgets and can't stay in their seat in the classroom displaying this behavior as a result of hyperactivity or a deficit in impulse control seen in ADHD, or is it due to a child feeling increasing discomfort in a particular social situation? Is the child who is not able to sustain attention during a task or not listening to directions a result of a deficit in attention span from ADHD or due to the fact that the child might be overly preoccupied with concern about passing as their affirmed gender? Or is it a result of both such as in Dana's case where her ability to focus seemed to be worsened after her disclosure of her transgender identity and was observed by her parents to be more self-occupied with her concern of passing and not being judged as "not being a real girl?" Thus, to address the clinical question #1—*To what extent can the clinician parse out the diagnostic complexities when assessing a child with gender identity concerns presenting with ADHD symptomatology*—the following would be important to consider:

The psychiatrist plays a crucial role in educating parents that certain presenting symptoms (in this case, inattention and impulsivity) of a child with GD may be one of several possibilities: (1) mostly related to the underlying gender issue, in which case the symptoms would resolve by solely addressing the gender dysphoria; (2) related to both the gender issue and potentially another diagnosis (or more), in which case both issues need to be addressed; (3) and if the latter is true, there may or may not be an interplay between the gender nonconformity and the other diagnoses (in this case, impulsivity may have affected Dana's potential premature disclosure to other children about her identity). To elaborate further, there are children with gender-related issues (either gender nonconformity and/or gender dysphoria) with co-occurring ADHD where the ADHD symptoms are assumed to be purely a manifestation of the gender issue. Then there are children who present with both a gender identity-related concern *and* ADHD (or some other disorder). Or there may be children where ADHD is the primary concern and gender nonconformity might be mistakenly assessed to be gender dysphoria by parents or others. Teasing these issues out might involve a slow titration of interventions to help clarify diagnoses and inform subsequent treatment recommendations.

In Dana's case there was evidence of the core symptoms of inattention and hyperactivity that persisted throughout different settings both prior to and after she made a social transition as female, which further led to the support of the diagnosis of ADHD in addition to gender dysphoria, as opposed to explaining some of the behavioral symptoms as a sequela from the distress of her gender dysphoria. In the event that Dana had presented to the clinic as Daniel (prior to social gender transition), it would not have been out of the question for Dana's parents to have assumed that Dana's inattention and impulsivity were related to a lack of gender transition, thus potentially prompting them to push for a social gender transition. Other parents may have wanted for ADHD symptomatology to be addressed first. The psychiatrist can help navigate these complex decisions by starting with less invasive interventions and measuring response, as one would do with any other child presenting with more than one issue at hand.

Addressing clinical question #2—*For prepubertal children with co-occurring ADHD and GD, what are the potential implications that the provider and parent must take into account when considering a social gender transition for that child?* The following could be understood from this clinical case presentation. There was also the presence of some oppositionality in the history of Dana. One of the most marked symptoms that parents saw in Dana was the tendency to actively defy adult requests and deliberately doing things that annoy others. Dana did not have other signs that could be seen with oppositional defiant disorder, such as being described as angry or resentful, being spiteful or vindictive, being easily annoyed by others, blaming others for her mistakes, losing her temper, or being argumentative with adults. In this case, much of the defiance that was seen was very much in relationship to rules the parents set up regarding how Dana presented and expressed her gender out of concern for her safety and wanting to protect her from the teasing and bullying she experienced in her previous community. Interestingly, with the compounding factor of carrying an ADHD diagnosis, it is reasonably possible that Dana was not deliberately trying to defy her parents' rules but may have lacked the level of impulse control to inhibit her expressions, thus resulting in evoking negative reactions from her peers. A primary goal of the parents was the hope that Dana would become more comfortable with who she is and not feel ashamed of her gender identity. The recommendation to engage in the child play group was to provide a safe space for children to socialize without the fear of stigma with both other children who are gender nonconforming and those who are not, since siblings were invited to the group as well.

Providing psychoeducation to the parents regarding the potential benefits and challenges of a social gender transition in a prepubertal child—regardless of the presence of a co-occurring diagnosis—would be important. An individualized approach that factors in the biopsychosocial circumstances of the child and family would help the family appreciate the complexities that a social gender transition may or may not have with respect to the child's emotional, psychological, and social functioning. Even in situations where parents may have already made the decision for their child to transition socially to another gender before an assessment, educating them on the current scientific understanding of the trajectories of these children would be useful. Helping the parents remain open to the possibility that the child may, in fact, not express this identity at a point later in time is important to convey so as to remove any element of coercion that the child may feel. This may sometimes be difficult for parents to hear, considering tolerating the ambiguity of the future is often not an easy task for parents to take on—whether it be about gender or any other aspect of their child's life.

For the child with oppositionality and/or ADHD symptoms, reconfiguring parental expectations about what a child is or is not able to do on a developmental level adds an entirely new layer of complexity. For example, well-intentioned parents may want to shield their child from the stigma of being gender nonconforming. Many parents choose to transition their children to another gender when gender dysphoria is apparent. However, an impulsive and/or inattentive child already is at risk for social ostracism and/or difficulty navigating trust and social interactions. Therefore, what might seem to be a reasonable intervention at the time (e.g., social gender transition) might actually create more challenges than the parents may have anticipated. There could be a conflicting message to the child: "we will support you to live authentically, however do not tell anyone because you will be made fun of." How this message is framed to the child, and whether or not the child can incorporate it in a way that is not shameful (e.g., "we love you for who you are, will love you if you change in the future, and let's discuss what is private [versus secret] for you"), is important to consider for the child.

These issues are also related to clinical question #3—*How does the combination of ADHD and gender dysphoria impact a child's social development or sense of self?* Clinically, there is a spectrum of ways that children with gender dysphoria share, disclose, or express their gender identity. Some children live their lives as their affirmed gender without sharing with others the details about their transition, whereas other children may very openly share with others these details. Often times the latter may be the case, when a child wants to socially transition, and there may be questions from peers or others who have known the child as their birth-assigned gender. In Dana's case, her parents had hoped the timing of their move to a new location would result in being able to avoid some of the teasing and bullying they experienced when she first transitioned by only telling those individuals that they felt needed to know (such as the school principal, scout troop leader, or very trusted family adult friends). Despite discussing with Dana the plan to not tell others that she is "transgender," Dana did end up telling some peers about her gender identity, only to find some negative reactions from peers who did not fully understand what being transgender meant. It was clear that Dana did not want to experience the teasing and bullying that she previously went through, so one must wonder if her disclosure was a result of being more impulsive and not thinking through the possible risk of telling others her gender identity or if this arose from Dana just wanting to fully express who she is as a person and not feel that she needed to hide certain aspects or details about herself.

Over time, Dana seemed to be much more focused on ensuring that others see her as being female. She has not further shared with other peers that she identifies as transgender, yet the degree to which she has internalized shame about feeling female yet being born with male anatomy is only something that can be known over time. Further support in both individual therapy and our play group may help Dana better manage situations where she may not get an accepting response, as well as potentially address the possible evolving conflict in Dana between wanting to tell others details about her true self and also wanting to keep some of those details private in order to avoid being teased or bullied.

Conclusion

Children with gender dysphoria and ADHD raise a number of questions in regard to how providers evaluate and work with them in alleviating the distress and behavioral issues that are often found. Both conditions lend themselves to having an impact on a child's emotional and social functioning and may lead to difficulties in how they communicate and interact with their peers. Decisions that are often made regarding how and when a child expresses their gender may be more complicated when families want to limit disclosure or expression in all settings in an effort to protect their child from negative responses, such as bullying. Various approaches in working with children with gender dysphoria are being utilized, but more understanding about the implications of how different approaches may impact this subset of children that carry diagnoses of ADHD and/or disruptive behavior disorders is needed. General approaches of continuing to show support and acceptance for the child's gender identity and expression, as well as providing additional support for both the child and family through individual and group therapeutic settings to help manage difficult situations surrounding social interactions, appeared to have been helpful. More research is needed in understanding how these conditions may interact and impact a child's well-being, as well as how we manage children with both conditions.

References

1. Steensma TD, Cohen-Kettenis PT. Gender transitioning before puberty? Arch Sex Behav. 2011;40:649–50. https://doi.org/10.1007/s10508-011-9752-2.
2. Olson K, Durwood L, DeMeueles M, McLaughlin K. Mental health of transgender children who are supported in their identities. Pediatrics. 2016;137(3):e20153223.
3. Steensma TD, McGuire JK, Kreukels BP, Beekman AJ, Cohen-Kettenis PT. Factors associated with desistence and persistence of childhood gender dysphoria: a quantitative follow-up study. J Am Acad Child Adolesc Psychiatry. 2013;52:582–90.
4. Edwards-Leeper L, Leibowitz S, Sangganjanavanich F. Affirmative practice with transgender and gender nonconforming youth: expanding the model. Psychol Sex Orientat Gend Divers. 2016;3(2):165–72.
5. Cohen-Kettenis PT, Owen A, Kaijser VG, Bradley SJ, Zuker KJ. Demographic characteristics, social competence, and behavior problems in children with gender identity disorder; a cross-national, cross-clinic comparative analysis. J Abnorm Child Psychol. 2003;31(1):41–53.
6. Wallien MS, Swaab H, Cohen-Kettenis PC. Psychiatric comorbidity among children with gender identity disorder. J Am Acad Child Adolesc Psychiatry. 2007;46(10):1307–14.
7. De Vries AL, Doreleijers TA, Steensma TD, Cohen-Kettenis PC. Psychiatric comorbidity in gender dysphoric adolescents. J Child Psychol Psychiatry. 2011;52(11):1195–202.
8. Strang JF, Kenworthy L, Dominska A, Sokoloff J, Kenealy LE, Berl M, et al. Increased gender variance in autism spectrum disorders and attention deficit hyperactivity disorder. Arch Sex Behav. 2014;43(8):1525–33.
9. Steensma TD, Zucker KJ, Kreukels BPC, VanderLaan DP, Wood H, Fuentes A, et al. Behavioral and emotional problems on the Teacher's Report Form: a cross-national, cross-clinic comparative analysis of gender dysphoric children and adolescents. J Abnorm Child Psychol. 2014;42:635–47.
10. Hoza B, Mrug S, Gerdes AC, Hinshaw SP, Bukowski WM, Gold JA, et al. What aspects of peer relationships are impaired in children with attention deficit hyperactivity disorder? J Consult Clin Psychol. 2005;73(3):411–23.
11. Hoza B. Peer functioning in children with ADHD. J Pediatr Psychol. 2007;32(6):655–63.
12. Humphreys K, Galan CA, Tottenham N, Lee S. Impaired social decision-making mediates the association between ADHD and social problems. J Abnorm Child Psychol. 2016;44:1023–32.

Chapter 8
Gender Dysphoria and Autism Spectrum Disorders

Aron Janssen

Introduction

Sitting across from me in my office was a 13-year-old, here for a consultation while home from his residential treatment center with a request from his family on how best to understand and support his continued insistence that he be allowed to wear dresses and be referred to as a girl. Over the years of previous treatments, he's been diagnosed with many things—intellectual disability (IQ of 55), autism, and bipolar disorder—but none of these labels do anything to accurately describe this ebullient youngster who deftly differentiates between internal experience and external expectations of gender. In answering my request to draw a self-portrait, his response was "Should I draw it as I see myself or how others see me?" As the evaluation proceeded, it raised several important questions: How do we understand gender identity development in someone with intellectual disability and an autism spectrum disorder? How do we differentiate between symptoms of autism (including intense, restricted interests) and symptoms of gender dysphoria? How do we assess an individual's ability to understand the irreversible effects of medical and surgical interventions? Utilizing this patient's experience, we will review the literature into the overlap between autism and gender dysphoria and discuss the unique considerations when working with kids that experience both. Please note, for the sake of the case discussion, this patient used both "he/him" and "she/her" pronouns at various points during our work together. The pronouns used will reflect the patient's preference at the time.

A. Janssen, MD
Department of Child and Adolescent Psychiatry, NYU Langone Health, NYU Child Study Center, New York, NY, USA
e-mail: aron.janssen@nyumc.org

A. Janssen, S. Leibowitz (eds.), *Affirmative Mental Health Care for Transgender and Gender Diverse Youth*, https://doi.org/10.1007/978-3-319-78307-9_8

Brief Literature Review

Autism spectrum disorders (ASDs) are a set of neurodevelopmental disorders that are defined by deficits in two major domains. The first domain encompasses persistent deficits in social communication and interaction across multiple contexts. This could include difficulties in social-emotional reciprocity (i.e., difficulty with back and forth conversation), difficulties in nonverbal communication used for the purpose of social interaction (i.e., maintaining eye contact, using gestures, etc.), or difficulties in understanding complex social relationships. The second domain encompasses restricted and repetitive patterns of behavior, interests, or activities. This could include repetitive motor movements or speech (i.e., echolalia, frequent lining up of toys or rocking back and forth), an inflexible adherence to routines, interests that are highly fixated and abnormal in intensity or focus, or hyper- or hyporeactivity to sensory input [1]. Symptoms from both domains must be present in the early developmental period and must lead to significant impairments in functioning. The American Academy of Pediatrics recommends that all children should be screened for ASD during well doctor visits at 1.5 and 2 years of age. There are a number of available screening and diagnostic instruments and interviews available that have evidence-based support for their use in children suspected to have autism [2]. For children suspected to have an ASD, a further evaluation consisting of a parent/caregiver interview and an observational assessment should be employed to ensure the accuracy of the diagnosis.

Gender dysphoria, which has been described in depth earlier in this book, is defined primarily by a persistent incongruence between one's assigned sex at birth and expressed/experienced gender [1]. Over the last decade, there has been increased evidence to suggest an association between gender dysphoria, gender variance, and ASDs [3–6]. Current literature suggests a bidirectional relationship; that is, individuals presenting with gender dysphoria are more likely to have a co-occurring diagnosis of ASD, and individuals presenting with a diagnosis of ASD are more likely to have a co-occurring diagnosis of gender dysphoria. Current prevalence rates for ASD in the general population range from 0.3 to 1.16% [7], and individuals with ASDs are approximately seven times more likely to be gender variant than same aged peers [3, 5].

Gender dysphoria, gender variance, and ASDs are complex phenomena that are present among all populations of varying degrees of expression. Given their frequent overlap, researchers have sought to understand possible common shared etiologic mechanisms. Some have theorized a role for genetics, prenatal exposure to hormones, or even environmental toxins [8, 9], but these theories are speculative at best. Given the lack of research into the known mechanisms for social and gender identity development, we are left to use clinical observation to reflect on similarities and dissimilarities between those with autism, those with gender variance, and those with both.

Case reports on individuals with gender dysphoria and autism have pointed to unique presentations and treatment implications. Individuals with both gender dysphoria and an ASD will commonly present with preoccupations that shape their life experiences, and this preoccupation may overlap with thinking about gender identity [10]. Furthermore, others have found that children with more profound intellectual disability, which frequently is present in children with ASDs, have more difficulty in establishing and articulating a gender identity that is consistent over time [11]. Jacobs et al. [12] discussed the role of impaired theory of mind and intolerance of ambiguity in shaping therapeutic interventions for individuals with both gender dysphoria and ASDs. These authors make a point to note that while there are unique elements to the individuals with autism and gender dysphoria, these unique elements should not be barriers to seeking out gender affirmative care.

In fact, the opposite is often the case. It is common for individuals with ASDs to have more difficulty in accessing transition-related care. Many practitioners are uncomfortable in assessing and/or working with individuals with both gender dysphoria and ASDs, and there is very limited pool of providers that have expertise (or even experience) with both. As such, individuals often face fragmented care with multiple different providers providing multiple different components to a treatment plan. However, for those of us lucky enough to work with this population, the rewards are self-evident, and there is a tremendous amount to learn by partnering with our patients to better understand their needs and experience.

Diagnosis and Assessment

JM was born to a biological mother with a history of schizophrenia and polysubstance abuse, and she was known to have used multiple substances during the pregnancy. JM was born on time, via vaginal delivery. He was born with typical male genitalia and had otherwise typical development. There was initial opiate withdrawal after birth; otherwise, the immediate postnatal period was unremarkable. JM was given up for adoption and placed with a foster family that later adopted him. His fine and gross motor skills were delayed, and he didn't say his first word until age 3 and didn't speak in full sentences until age 5. He would be noted to frequently flap his hands, rock back and forth, and would often do the same physical task over and over again. He was identified for early intervention and was diagnosed with autism and referred for intensive treatment.

Notably, by age 3, JM began demonstrating a clear preference for more typical feminine play. JM was preferentially drawn to dolls and his mother's clothes and shoes. While there was little demonstrated interest in socializing with other children, he was more attracted to the games played by the girls in his parents' social circles. As he got older, he began to play dress up, and his father recalled how JM's face would light up when he was allowed to wear a very specific pink tulle skirt. When the family asked about the significance of this preference, they were told that while some kids with autism are drawn to maps or trains or dinosaurs, JM was drawn to dresses.

By age 5, JM began to get aggressive. He would often appear to be internally preoccupied, and he would go days without more than an hour or 2 of sleep. He appeared in these periods to be even more drawn to dress up and to his mother's clothes and make up, and when these items were restricted from use, as was directed by his treatment providers, he would become increasingly agitated and would throw things around the house. And yet, when his mood was stabilized, and he was again sleeping through the night, he continued to have clear preference toward feminine attire and appearance. He would pee only from a sitting position and began to ask his parents when he would develop breasts. While he never made statements such as "I am a girl," he did discuss his belief that he would become a girl when he grew up.

Multiple evaluations and repeated neuropsychological testing was done, which consistently reinforced the intellectual disability, the autism, and the bipolar disorder. And at every step along the way, these were the reasons given for JM's longing for femininity. By the time he reached his teen years, JM has been living in a residential treatment facility for the past 2 years to manage his increasingly unsafe behaviors at home. While there, he began to assert requests to wear girls' clothing and go by a girls' name. His treatment center, working from the recommendations by his outpatient providers that this preference was a "restricted interest," disallowed him from accessing any feminine attire, and he was admonished when he requested to use a girls' name.

JM's parents, having seen a documentary about transgender children, wondered if they needed a different approach and brought him for an evaluation with a gender specialist. In this initial evaluation, it was clear that while JM certainly met criteria for ASD and for bipolar disorder, JM also had lifelong gender dysphoria and a female identity that had never been affirmed. During the initial meeting, JM was eager to tell his story and told me that he has always felt like a girl, that he hates "(his) twig," and wants to live full time as a girl. He told me in the initial meeting that he was sure of this, and his history was consistent. In every period of his life, in every mood state, JM was a child that consistently affirmed a female identity. However, his conception of gender was different than many of the kids I have seen. For example, JM reported that while he preferred a female name and attire, he did not mind he/him pronouns. He used he/him when referring to himself regardless of how he was presenting and which name he utilized. His experience of his gender was more about his own feeling and experience rather than how others saw him. He cared less about if he was perceived of as a girl than about whether he was allowed to wear what he wanted to wear and how he saw himself. So when I asked him to draw a picture of himself, of course I told him to draw it how he saw himself, which was as a princess in a ball gown with long, blonde hair.

Management

Given JM's clear gender dysphoria, we worked on a treatment plan to help JM manage the distress felt. First, the treatment center was educated on gender dysphoria and the role they can play in supporting JM in exploring identity rather than restricting such developmentally appropriate tasks. Next, we worked with JM and family on social transition. Over a period of several months, JM transitioned to going by a girls' name full time, wearing girls' clothes (as she saw them), and she began to use she/her pronouns throughout the various contexts in her life.

There were unique challenges posed because of her co-occurring ASD. For example, JM could not understand why she couldn't wear a ball gown in every context and had a hard time understanding why others in her life had a hard time in using her new name and affirmed pronouns. She didn't appear to be particularly bothered by this but more perplexed. She had made the transition—why was it that not everyone seemed to notice? She needed help in constructing her narrative of her experience—how could she help others to understand her process, thereby helping herself to understand how others may think and react in certain situations. She had to learn about safety, bathroom use, and personal boundaries in a way that was at times much more explicit than others require.

Given JM's intellectual disability and ASD, one of the challenges in our work was establishing how to assess her capacity to make decisions that lead to irreversible and partially irreversible challenges. Given her limitations, this required more concrete examples of the risks, benefits, and alternatives through use of photos and videos to aid in discussions. We involved JM's parents in these discussions, and thankfully JM had parents that were supportive and appreciated the improvements that JM made with social transition and were eager to support JM in her decisions in her care.

As treatment progressed, and puberty began in earnest, she was able to articulate very clearly the increase in distress as a result of her changing body and a wish for puberty suppression. At 16, she has been living her life as a girl for over 2½ years and is about to start estrogen.

Clinical Pearls and Pitfalls

JM was lucky to have a supportive family that had the means and the resources to seek out a second opinion regarding gender identity development and was able to access care that was affirming. This process had a profound positive effect on her life. However, it is easy to imagine that if JM's parents were less supportive, or if they lived in an area without access to a gender specialist, JM would still be living in an environment in which she was punished for asserting her identity as a girl. Access to affirming and effective care is a chronic problem for children with gender variance and even more so for children with gender variance and an ASD. Working with JM was a privilege, and JM was excited to know that her experience would help others like her. In discussing the case, there were several main points to review: implications for assessment and diagnosis, assessing an individual's ability to give consent, unique treatment implications, and ensuring access to care.

Diagnostically, individuals with ASDs often have intense restricted interests. For example, one of my patients with autism is obsessed with laundry soap. She knows every possible type of laundry soap, wants only to talk about laundry soap, and at any given time will have two to three different kinds of travel size laundry soap that she carries with her to smell and to show off. If given the opportunity, she will spend an entire conversation entirely dedicated to laundry soap. This obsessive interest though has developed over time. When she was younger, she was obsessed with hair and would play with her own hair so much that it would take an hour every night for her father to untangle it. Often this kind of restricted interests are used by those skeptical of gender dysphoria to dismiss a child's assertion of their own gender. For example, some might say: "My child wanted to be a horse when she was younger—we didn't allow her to identity as a horse then, so why when she says she now wants to be a boy would I allow that?" The reality is that there is a different developmental process for gender identity than for a child's normal imaginative process of trying on different personas and interests. And yet, for some children with ASDs, these interests are so intense they disallow for easy exploration of other more complex aspects of the self. This then begs the question—how do we understand if a transgender identity is authentic or a restricted interest? And does it matter?

One factor to look for is consistency of expression. For some individuals with ASD (particularly those who are nonverbal), it is difficult for them to easily communicate their needs and desires. As such, for some kids, these needs might be expressed like it was for JM with statements consistent with a transgender identity. For others, this may be frequent tantrums when forced to wear the clothes typical of their assigned sex at birth or a frequent repetitive play with more stereotypically masculine or feminine toys. For individuals with gender dysphoria, we would expect that as a child consolidates their gender identity, there would be a consistency across time and situations. For JM, this meant that she espoused a female identity when manic, when euthymic, and when depressed. She espoused it at home, at school, and in residential treatment. While the skeptics will use the horse example, I have yet to hear of a child that will consistently espouse an identity of that of a horse consistently over years with a worsening with puberty. As such, while identity development in more complex among children with ASDs, it does not mean that they cannot tell us what we need to know, if only we learn how to listen.

Another factor to help in the assessment is by examining the impact of various interventions on the individuals functioning and sense of self. For JM, many interventions were put into place over the years to attempt to in some way decondition the gender identity and expression. Most notably, JM had some behavioral difficulties at the residential treatment center, and their treatment plan included attempts to reduce more feminine expression. This was in context to time spent at home in which JM was allowed to dress as she wanted and was demonstrably more bright and cheerful during those times. Similarly, when the residential treatment center began to allow JM to assert her identity as a girl, use she/her pronouns, and dress in dresses, the behavioral difficulties diminished. She continued to struggle at times with her mood and her thought disorder persisted, but her overall functioning significantly improved with each step taken in her social transition.

Social transition represents a completely reversible intervention with very few risks. The risks involved are mostly situational and include potential exposure to bias and violence, which is important for the clinician and the family to address however possible. When considering the reversible and potentially irreversible interventions such as puberty blockers, cross sex hormones, and surgery, it is important to assess an individual's capacity to consent to these treatments. For JM, she had significant intellectual impairments; however, she spent much of her time looking at information around transition and had a surprising degree of knowledge of the risks of the various interventions. This will not be the case for all individuals with ASDs. This places clinicians, families, and the patients themselves in a potential bind. How do we know how best to proceed when a patient lacks the means to communicate an understanding of the risks, benefits, and alternatives to a particular intervention?

In working with JM and her family, we are able to work collaboratively to discuss both in individual sessions and in family sessions all the various options, including hormones. We used verbal means and pictures online to review the various expected changes and the possible risks involved. For JM, despite her limitations, she was able to provide a clear assent, and her parents were able to provide consent for the various interventions. For most patients with psychiatric disorders, the capacity to consent is retained, even during active illness, and it is important to note that delayed access to transition-related care is correlated with worse outcomes for transgender individuals. While clearly the consent process is more complex with these individuals, it is possible nevertheless to engage patients in a shared decision-making process.

In treatment with individuals with both gender dysphoria and ASDs, it is important to take into account the unique considerations for each patient. For JM, the interventions around the gender dysphoria was one of the most straightforward pieces of the treatment plan. For others, it is much more complex. For example, some patients struggle with understanding the social cues that are associated with gender role. One patient I was working with could not understand why her transition went unnoticed, and we had to work for her to understand that since she had not changed anything about her appearance, pronoun, or name, it was difficult for others to know that she was not asserting herself as a woman. Another patient who struggled to communicate his needs spent several months in therapy having a difficult time engaging and only was able to engage in therapy after it was discovered that it was not the interpersonal aspect of the therapy that was uncomfortable (which had been the assumption) but instead the patient's discomfort about the sound of his voice. Discomfort in one's voice is a common occurrence in transgender individuals, but this individual patient had difficulties in social communication at baseline which made it difficult for him to express this in a way that felt safe.

Much of the treatment of gender dysphoria involves interacting with various systems—the healthcare system, the educational system, the family system, the legal system, and often individuals with ASDs need more assistance in advocating for their needs in these varied environments. Clinicians working with people with ASDs and gender dysphoria play an important role in this vital advocacy.

Conclusion

Individuals with ASDs are more likely to have gender dysphoria, and individuals with gender dysphoria are more likely to have an ASD. As more attention is given to this overlap, we will continue to discover the diverse ways in which gender is understood and expressed. Having a different view of gender development should not lead to disenfranchisement from treatment; however, having autism has historically been a barrier to accessing transition-related care. I would argue that individuals with autism can at times break down the artificiality of the rigidity of gender identity and expression more effectively than their non-autistic peers. When practitioners can learn to partner with their patients, we will recognize how much they can teach us about their experiences and, by extension, our own.

References

1. American Psychiatric Association. Diagnostic and statistical manual of mental disorders. 5th ed. Arlington, VA: American Psychiatric Publishing; 2013.
2. Huerta M, Lord C. Diagnostic evaluation of autism spectrum disorders. Pediatr Clin N Am. 2012;59(1):103–11.
3. Janssen A, Huang H, Duncan C. Gender variance among youth with autism spectrum disorders: a retrospective chart review. Transgender Health. 2016;1(1):63–8.
4. Van Schalkwyk G, Klingensmith K, Volkman F. Gender identity and autism spectrum disorders. Yale J Biol Med. 2015;88:81–3.
5. Strang J, Kenworthy L, Dominska A, Sokoloff J, Kenealy LE, Berl M, et al. Increased gender variance in autism spectrum disorders and attention deficit hyperactivity disorder. Arch Sex Behav. 2014;43:1525–33.
6. de Vries A, Noens I, Cohen-Kettenis P, van Berckelaer-Onnes IA, Doreleijers TA. Autism spectrum disorders in gender dysphoric children and adolescents. J Autism Dev Disord. 2010;40:930–6.
7. Eisabbagh M, Divan G, Koh YS, Kim YS, Kauchali S, Marcín C, et al. Global prevalence of autism and other pervasive developmental disorders. Autism Res. 2012;5:160–79.
8. Bejerot S, Humble MB, Gardner A. Endocrine disruptors, the increase of autism spectrum disorder and its comorbidity with gender identity disorder—a hypothetical association. Int J Androl. 2011;34(5:Pt. 2):e350.
9. Swan SH, Liu F, Hines M, Kruse RL, Wang C, Redmon JB, et al. Prenatal phthalate exposure and reduced masculine play in boys. Int J Androl. 2010;33:259–69.
10. Williams PG, Allard AM, Sears L. Case study: cross-gender preoccupations with two male children with autism. J Autism Dev Disord. 1996;26:635–42.
11. Lee A, Hobson RP. On developing self-concepts: a controlled study of children and adolescents with autism. J Child Psychol Psychiatry. 1998;39:1131–44.
12. Jacobs L, Rachlin K, Erickson-Schroth L, Janssen A. Gender dysphoria and co-occurring autism spectrum disorders: review, case examples and treatment considerations. LGBT Health. 2014;1:277–82.

Chapter 9
Anxiety and Gender Dysphoria

Laura Edwards-Leeper

Case Introduction

Presenting Concern

Alex (given name: Alexandra), a 15-year-old birth-assigned female, presented to a clinical psychologist who specializes in working with transgender and gender non-conforming youth for an evaluation to better understand her gender identity and explore whether pursuing a medical intervention (testosterone) would be in her best interest. Alex's parents contacted her pediatrician after she came out to them, and the pediatrician referred Alex for a psychological/gender evaluation. Alex uses female pronouns but shared with her parents 1 month ago that she identifies herself as a boy. Alex has not taken any steps toward socially transitioning. In addition to gender dysphoria, Alex presents with significant anxiety that results in a sense of overwhelming fear, particularly in social situations. Alex experiences panic attacks as well. Alex shared with her parents via text message that she wants to start testosterone treatment and have her breasts removed, but she is resistant to talking with them about this. As a result, Alex's parents wonder if she is "making this up," and "just trying to get attention."

Clinical Relevance

This case addresses the following four important questions relevant to Alex's clinical care:

L. Edwards-Leeper, PhD
School of Graduate Psychology, Pacific University, Hillsboro, OR, USA
e-mail: laura.edwards-leeper@pacificu.edu

A. Janssen, S. Leibowitz (eds.), *Affirmative Mental Health Care for Transgender and Gender Diverse Youth*, https://doi.org/10.1007/978-3-319-78307-9_9

1. For adolescent gender diverse patients presenting with significant anxiety and requesting hormone treatment, how well controlled should the anxiety be prior to starting medical treatment for the potential gender dysphoria?
2. How important is it for adolescent gender diverse patients to explore the ways in which their anxiety may and may not be related to their gender dysphoria, and how much of this exploration should occur prior to the youth starting hormonal intervention?
3. Is it reasonable to expect adolescent gender diverse patients to undergo some degree of social transition prior to the initiation of irreversible medical interventions?
4. How important is it for time to be spent with parents of gender diverse patients to hear and validate their concerns and provide education and support prior to the adolescent beginning medical interventions?

Literature Review

Research indicates that many transgender youth experience heightened levels of depression and anxiety, among other mental health diagnoses, upon first being seen in a gender clinic [1]. A recent study utilizing a chart review methodology found that transgender patients (ages 12–29) were more likely to report anxiety and depression than their cisgender peers, as well as engage in self-harm, suicidal ideation, and prior attempts [2]. Similarly, researchers examining results obtained from formal psychological instruments used during comprehensive evaluations with transgender youth discovered that 39% of the youth had clinically elevated internalizing scores and 48% were in the clinically elevated range by parent report [3]. Additionally, 24% of these youth reported suicidal ideation. This study also found a positive correlation between anxiety and age, such that older transgender adolescents reported more anxiety than younger transgender adolescents.

Although these studies highlight the negative mental health experiences of many transgender youth, intervening medically has been shown to improve these experiences with many of the youth. Dutch researchers have found that most appropriately screened transgender adolescents who are offered puberty-blocking medication do remarkably well in regard to their mental health, often displaying symptoms comparable to their same-age cisgender peers [4]. The assumed reasons for this positive outcome are related to the benefits of the puberty-blocking medication. First, it buys more time for the adolescent to further explore their gender identity without the added stress of secondary sex characteristics that are not aligned with their affirmed gender identity. Second, because the puberty suppression medication prevents the development of secondary sex characteristics, the individual is more likely to be perceived by others as their affirmed gender when starting gender-affirming hormone treatment, if that is their goal [5].

Unfortunately, many transgender youth do not present to healthcare providers during the early stages of puberty; thus, they do not reap the full benefit of this intervention. It is believed that a reason for elevated mental health symptoms among transgender adolescents is in part due to their severe gender dysphoria that is exacerbated by having anatomical features that are incongruent with their affirmed gender, along with the social stigma and rejection that many of these youth face [6]. This is often exacerbated when they complete the irreversible puberty of a gender with which they do not identify. However, parents and providers may wonder if the gender identity concern is a symptom of the youth's mental health struggles, rather than a factor contributing to their poor mental health. This can lead to heightened concern by parents regarding starting irreversible medical interventions for their troubled teenager, and providers may sometimes share this concern. Although this is a valid point and must be taken seriously during the evaluation process, it is equally important to recognize the critical role of parental support for the mental health of their transgender children. Ryan et al. found that gender and sexual minority youth who have the support of their parents show resiliency in both physical and mental health domains [7]. Similarly, a recent study found that young transgender children who were supported by their parents in their affirmed gender showed similar levels of depressive symptoms and only slightly elevated anxiety as compared to their cisgender counterparts [8].

In summary, although many researchers have shown that transgender youth often experience increased mental health symptoms, specifically related to anxiety and depression, this appears to be more likely when they are not able to obtain the medical and mental health services they need. Research suggests that youth who are evaluated and supported by mental health providers and are supported with social transition and/or medical intervention when appropriate are incredibly resilient and do not exhibit elevated levels of depression and anxiety. There is also a dearth of research on the relationship between social anxiety and gender dysphoria in transgender youth. Given the social concerns present for many transgender individuals related to being misgendered, judged, and potentially harassed, one could hypothesize that a positive correlation exists between gender dysphoria and symptoms of social anxiety.

Case Report

History of Presenting Concern

Alex, a 15-year-old birth-assigned female, presented with her parents for a comprehensive gender evaluation. Alex stated that she was hoping to start testosterone treatment as soon as possible because she "felt like a guy." Alex also reported significant anxiety, for which she was not being treated. Alex reported that she always felt "on edge" and worried "about everything." She explained that her anxiety was worse at school because she worried what people were thinking about her, often feeling as if peers were talking about and laughing at her. Alex also reported that she was afraid to speak in class, mostly because of her feminine voice. Alex reported feeling anxious since age 12, around the time when puberty started. At that time, Alex explained that she had a difficult time fitting in with her female peers and became self-conscious about her body.

Alex's parents confirmed that Alex started becoming more anxious around age 12 but indicated that she had always been an "overly sensitive" and "slow-to-warm-up" child. They shared that as a child, Alex typically focused exclusively on one friend at a time. Alex's parents shared that many of Alex's peers identified as transgender and gender fluid, and they worried that she was glomming on to this identity as a way of trying to fit in.

Relevant Psychiatric History

Alex's parents reported that Alex experienced separation anxiety when younger, becoming inconsolable whenever she was dropped off at daycare. This resulted in Alex's mother quitting her job so that she could be at home with Alex. They further reported that Alex was diagnosed with obsessive compulsive disorder (OCD) at age 7, due to excessive handwashing and ritualistic behaviors that she felt compelled to perform before going to bed every night. Alex was seen by a psychologist to address the OCD, and parents reported that these behaviors significantly improved by the time Alex was 10 years old.

Alex shared that she had felt anxious for as long as she could remember but that it became significantly worse around age 12, when puberty started. She also reported that her anxiety made it difficult for her to be happy as a child, and she recalled her parents and teachers often asking if she was "okay." Parents confirmed this, stating that Alex often had a serious or slightly concerned look on her face as a child. When puberty started, Alex stated that she became very self-conscious about her body and was sometimes teased for being overweight. For approximately 1 year (ages 12–13), she reported engaging in non-suicidal self-injurious behavior on her forearms several times per week, which she reported was tied to her anxiety. Alex's parents connected her with a therapist when they realized that she was cutting herself, and she was also referred to a psychiatrist at that time for a medication evaluation. Alex saw this therapist for approximately 1 year. Alex was started on fluoxetine to address the anxiety, but due to side effects (dizziness and stomachaches), she discontinued the medication after 4 months. Alex denied any cutting behavior in the last 9 months, stating that she was tired of her mother getting on her case about it.

Relevant Gender Development History

When exploring early childhood gender history, Alex reported being a fairly "typical girl" when younger, playing with Barbie dolls, dressing up in princess dresses, watching Strawberry Shortcake cartoons, and decorating her room in pink and purple. She reported that she wore mostly clothing that would be considered gender neutral but did not mind wearing dresses. Alex stated that she never really thought about her body when younger, not desiring a male body or having any strong feelings about her female anatomy. Alex further reported that she never thought about whether she would grow up to be a man/woman or a mother/father when she was younger but did experience some fear about growing up in general. Alex reported feeling as if something was not "right" with her during first grade, when she had a hard time connecting with her female peers. She stated that she thought about trying to play with the boys but was too shy to approach them. Alex's parents reported that Alex was a very "typical" girl through elementary school. They confirmed Alex's report regarding her more feminine interests and toy preferences. They added that Alex always chose stereotypical feminine Halloween costumes and participated in ballet for several years when younger.

Alex reported that it was not until approximately 9 months ago when she realized that she felt more like a boy than a girl. She explained that she was unaware of transgender people prior to that time. Alex reported seeing a television show that had a transgender man on it and realized that experience/identity fit for her. Soon after, she met a peer at school who identified as nonbinary. Alex reported that this friend talked with her and helped her realize that she was transgender. Alex started doing research on the Internet, and as she learned more about transgender individuals, her dysphoria became worse until she eventually realized that she had to come out to her parents. Alex shared that she texted her parents several weeks ago and told them that she felt like a boy. She said that her parents were trying to be supportive but seemed skeptical. Alex stated that her parents kept asking her questions, which was increasing her anxiety and causing her to shut down emotionally.

Alex's parents stated that even into puberty, Alex seemed like a typical preteen girl in their opinion. For example, they reported that she experimented with makeup, wore girls' clothing, and reported having crushes on boys. Parents stated that around age 13, Alex became increasingly depressed and started hanging out with her peers who were into "dark things." They stated that she started wearing mostly black, stayed in her room most of the time, and started cutting herself. Parents reported that Alex appeared less feminine during this time, but it was not until approximately 9 months ago that she came out to them as transgender. Parents reported that they were extremely shocked by this news, given the lack of apparent gender dysphoria in her history. They reported that they are trying to be supportive but that they are skeptical. Parents shared that Alex has always been very impressionable and easily influenced by peers, often out of a desire to feel accepted. Parents explained that they are worried that Alex's current identification as transgender may be a result of feeling depressed and anxious, and finding some peer acceptance among the gender and sexual minority students at her school.

When assessing the development of gender-related body dysphoria, Alex further reported that the changes in her body during puberty were distressing for her, primarily because she gained weight. Alex explained that she was teased about her weight when younger, so the increased weight gain at puberty was very difficult for her. Alex shared that she was not happy about breast development and tried to hide her breasts by wearing loose fitting clothing. She reported that she hated wearing a bra but would often wear a sports bra to try to flatten her chest. Alex stated that menstruation was "annoying and painful" but stated that it was not overly distressing. In reflecting back about Alex's reaction to her body changing in puberty, Alex's parents reported that breast development seemed somewhat upsetting to Alex, but they did not recall it being as upsetting as what Alex reported. They recalled that Alex did not want to purchase "typical" bras but only wanted to wear sports bras at that time. Alex's parents noticed her becoming more self-conscious about her body during early puberty, but they assumed this was due to weight gain. They further shared that menstruation seemed uneventful for Alex from their perspective.

Alex reported that her gender dysphoria has progressively increased and that she feels the only thing that will alleviate her distress is testosterone treatment and top surgery. Alex stated that if she could choose, she would have top surgery first, as her chest was the most upsetting aspect of her body currently. She reported that she had not socially transitioned because she was too anxious to do so, worrying that people would misgender her if she did not appear more masculine and have a deeper voice. Alex reported that she was unlikely to pursue bottom surgery in the future, as this was not important to her.

In regard to Alex's expectations for testosterone treatment, she indicated that she mostly wanted a deeper voice. She was less interested in increased body and facial hair, stating that she would likely shave her hair if it was too irritating. Alex was less familiar with other effects of testosterone, such as increased libido, acne, and clitoral enlargement. She indicated feeling generally "fine" about these additional possible changes. When asked about her thoughts about future fertility, Alex reported that she would "just adopt," because being pregnant seemed physically painful.

Psychosocial Factors

Alex lives with her biological mother, father, and 11-year-old brother. She reported being unsure how her brother feels about her gender identity and stated that she has never been close to him. She explained that she has tried to avoid him recently because he has started male puberty and it makes her jealous. She reported that she often lashes out at her brother verbally because of this. Alex's parents confirmed that Alex and her brother have never gotten along well. They stated that Alex had a difficult time when her brother was born and always seemed jealous that he made friends more easily and had a closer relationship with their father.

Alex describes her race as Caucasian and reported that her family does not report any strong ethnic ties. Alex's immediate family is not religious, but the extended family on both sides identifies as Christian. Alex's mother's family is more conservative and Alex reported feeling that they may not be accepting of her male identity. Alex expressed some concern about the possible extended family members' reactions, as she had been close to her extended family on her mother's side when younger, particularly her grandmother. Alex's family identified their socioeconomic status as middle class. Her father is a high school math teacher, and her mother is a nurse.

Alex is a sophomore in high school, although she often misses school due to her anxiety. Alex and her parents are considering switching her to online schooling to help minimize this added stress. Alex received average grades during elementary and middle school, but her grades have deteriorated in the last 2 years. Alex reported difficulty focusing in class and often forgetting to turn in her homework. Alex has never had an Individualized Education Plan, been held back, or skipped a grade. Alex reported a plan to attend community college after high school and indicated that she was interested in pursuing graphic art.

Alex had not come out about her male identity at school and had not thought about how to talk to the school about making a social transition. Alex's parents were confused by this, as they feel that this lack of a plan on Alex's part suggests that she is not truly serious about being transgender. Alex indicated that the school seems to be accepting of transgender and gender fluid students, as she is aware of a transgender student who is allowed to use the nurse's bathroom.

Alex reported having two friends, one of whom identifies as a transboy and the other identifies as genderqueer. Alex indicated that she does not spend time with these friends outside of school but does interact with them via text messaging and social media. Alex indicated that her sexual orientation is asexual and that she is panromantic. For Alex, this means that she does not experience sexual feelings, may be interested in having a romantic relationship in the future, and the gender identity of the individual does not matter to her. Alex was surprised to learn that testosterone treatment may increase her libido, and she was unsure if this would be a welcome change. For fun, Alex enjoys cosplay, watching YouTube videos and Netflix, and listening to music.

Mental Status Exam

Alex presented to the evaluation appointment dressed in gender neutral clothing (jeans, flannel shirt, and converse shoes), wore her hair in androgynous style, and displayed gender neutral mannerisms and voice. She appeared very anxious for the first 30 min of the appointment, which was evidenced by her leg shaking, poor eye contact, and hesitancy when responding to questions. Alex appeared more comfortable as the evaluation continued and gradually became more forthcoming. Alex reported that her mood was "anxious" most of the time. Her affect during the appointment was fairly flat, although it became more appropriately animated when she shared her interest in cosplay. Alex's insight and judgment appeared fair. There were no concerns regarding her thought process or content. She was cordial when interacting with her parents, although she was much quieter when they were in the room with her.

DSM Diagnoses

Based on the information obtained during the evaluation appointment, Alex met the criteria for gender dysphoria in adolescents/adults and generalized anxiety disorder. She was also given a provisional diagnosis of depressive disorder unspecified and social anxiety, as it was unclear if the symptoms associated with these disorders were secondary to her gender dysphoria. A rule-out of attention deficit hyperactivity disorder (ADHD) was given due to her difficulty focusing and completing homework, although there was not enough information obtained during the clinical interview to make a definitive diagnosis.

Preliminary Biopsychosocial Formulation

Alex's presentation, which includes gender dysphoria, is considered complex for a number of reasons. First, neither Alex nor her parents reported a history of gender dysphoria for Alex in childhood, and in fact, they all indicated that Alex was a more stereotypical girl when younger. Although this detail does make the clinical picture more complex, it is not uncommon for transgender adolescents and adults to report their gender development to not include severe dysphoria in childhood [5].

Another aspect of this case that makes it more complex is the timing and way in which Alex described beginning to identify as male. Although it is common for dysphoria to intensify for transgender youth at the onset of puberty due to the distress caused by the development of secondary sex characteristics, Alex's distress at this developmental stage did not appear to be directly or solely tied to gender dysphoria, except for her breast development. Alex reported experiencing increased social ostracism during middle school and a history of being teased about her weight. She indicated more concern about breast development and very little about menstruation, which is often distressing for transgender boys and men.

Alex's parents reported she has always been an impressionable and easily influenced child, struggling to fit in with her peers. Given this history and reported personality trait, the fact that Alex started identifying as transgender after learning about it on television and then having a gender nonbinary friend help her realize that she was transgender is worth noting. It is possible that Alex is still in the midst of exploring this aspect of her identity. To adequately tease out the degree to which Alex's sought-after interventions are a result of an underlying core identity versus that of an undue external influence by peers, further exploration of the issue would be beneficial.

Alex is also struggling with fairly severe mental health concerns. Based on her self-report, the report of parents, and the results from the battery of psychological measures used in the evaluation, it is clear that Alex's anxiety and depressive symptoms are not being adequately treated. Additionally, she has a history of self-harm (and suicidal ideation), and possibly undiagnosed ADHD. Her parents reported a childhood diagnosis of OCD, and they shared a family psychiatric history positive for anxiety, depression, and bipolar disorder. Alex also has a younger brother who was diagnosed with high-functioning autism. Thus, in Alex's case, it is possible that her mental health symptoms have a biological underpinning and may not solely be the result of her gender dysphoria.

This case is also a bit more perplexing than some because although Alex states that she wants testosterone treatment and top surgery, she has not moved forward with any steps in the way of social transitioning. This is particularly interesting given that her parents have told her that they would support her in this, and the school would likely be supportive, per Alex. Without further exploration with Alex, we cannot be sure whether her decision to not socially transition is related to her degree of dysphoria, a fear of how others will treat her if she transitions, other anxiety related to her gender identity and reactions by others, or other factors. Given what we know about this case, it seems plausible that Alex's severe anxiety is the main reason for her being unable to move forward with a social transition. She stated that she feels that with the initiation of testosterone treatment, her anxiety will decrease and her confidence will improve enough to allow her to socially transition. However, it is also possible that her anxiety may increase upon starting testosterone, either as a direct result of the hormone itself or as a result of physical and/or social changes not meeting her expectations. For example, if Alex continues to be misgendered after starting testosterone, and/or if her anxiety does not significantly improve, she may become more distraught upon realizing that testosterone did not "fix" everything.

Additionally, it would be clinically negligent, given Alex's difficulty socially through childhood and adolescence, coupled with her mental health concerns and impressionable personality, at a developmental stage when peer influence is prevalent, to not consider the possibility that Alex's male identity is one part of her gender journey, but not the final destination. This is the concern that Alex's parents clearly articulated.

Finally, we must also consider whether Alex is able to provide informed consent for the medical intervention she is seeking. At the time of this evaluation, it was not clear whether Alex fully understood all of the potential effects of testosterone, and her consideration of the potential impact on her fertility was very limited. Alex's degree of insight into her identity and her understanding of what it means to be a man or a woman was also limited. The results from the gender measures used in the evaluation further indicated that while Alex endorsed gender dysphoria and identification as a boy, her responses suggested some uncertainty about this. Her responses on a body image measure further indicated that she was dissatisfied with every anatomical feature listed, not just those that are specific to her female anatomy. If she does not adequately understand her identity and the implications of the body-altering medical intervention she is considering, the risk of her later regretting the decision in the future increases.

Treatment Course

Treatment for Alex was multipronged, involving individual therapy, therapy including her parents, working with the school, referring for psychopharmacological intervention, and encouraging involvement with a community transgender support group. Additionally, meeting with a pediatric endocrinologist was recommended. Each of these will be described in some detail.

It was recommended that Alex reconnect with a mental health provider who was knowledgeable about both gender identity issues common among teenagers and treatment for anxiety and depression. In many cases, providers are comfortable with one, but not both, of these elements. In this case, the evaluating psychologist assisted the family with identifying an appropriate provider. The focus of treatment was on Alex's severe anxiety symptoms with the use of empirically supported treatments (cognitive behavioral therapy, including exposure treatment), but with a particular sensitivity to the ways in which the gender issue exacerbated the symptoms. As a result of this added piece, the interventions often needed to be adjusted to remain culturally sensitive and effective. For example, given that much of Alex's social anxiety was due to her voice being higher than a typical male's, her therapy goals did not require her to engage in a traditional exposure exercise, which might have involved openly talking more in class. Instead, other aspects of Alex's social anxiety were addressed, such as encouraging her to get out of the house and attend a transgender support group. This provided her with a safe place in which she could build her confidence and begin to interact with her peers to help overcome her social anxiety.

The work with Alex's mental health provider also assisted her with developing a plan and gaining confidence to slowly take steps in her social transition. The benefit of doing this prior to starting a medical intervention was to give Alex the opportunity to "try out" openly living and presenting as a male while having the space to process this experience in therapy, prior to initiating irreversible medical interventions that would permanently change her body. Alex was encouraged to take slow steps in this direction, starting by wearing male clothing and using her preferred name and pronouns in the safety of her own home and possibly in the company of close friends. She was then encouraged to experiment with this in safe places outside of the home, such as when meeting with her therapist and when attending a transgender support group. Eventually Alex was encouraged to go to public places where she felt confident she would not see people she knew (given that this was one of her initial fears in presenting as male in public), such as when her family was on vacation.

Alex's treatment also involved working with her parents. Specifically, the evaluating psychologist provided education, validation, and support to Alex's parents when they first shared their perspective on Alex's gender concerns during the comprehensive evaluation. Alex's parents were then included in some aspects of her ongoing therapy, when the therapist felt this would be worthwhile. For example, when Alex gained the confidence to start making steps in her social transition, the therapist met with Alex and her parents to discuss the plan and to ensure that they would support her. Additionally, because Alex's mother was having a particularly difficult time with grief and loss issues (i.e., grieving the loss of the daughter she thought she had and the future she imagined for Alex), she was referred to her own therapist who was also knowledgeable about transgender youth and the typical experiences of parents going through the process of having a child transition.

The school was also invited to play a role in helping Alex through this process, which was accomplished by both the therapist and Alex's parents advocating for her in the school system. For example, the school administrators were educated on the importance of providing restrooms inclusive of all genders, or at the very least allowing Alex to use the staff bathroom if she so desired. Additionally, arrangements were made for Alex to change clothing for her physical education class in the staff bathroom. The school was also encouraged to allow Alex to change her name in the system when she decided to do this, even though she had not legally changed her name. This is often important for transgender youth so that teacher (or more often substitute teachers) do not use the wrong name and pronouns.

Given that Alex's anxiety was so impairing, it was also recommended that she be evaluated by a child psychiatrist to determine if incorporating medication again to address her psychiatric symptoms would be worthwhile. In this case, it was determined that the medication would likely provide relief from the anxiety. Additionally, the response to the medication may itself provide important clues as to the degree to which the underlying gender dysphoria is a result of, or a separate issue from, the anxiety. Alex and her parents agreed to this recommendation.

Alex was also encouraged to attend a local transgender support group for additional support. This group served several purposes: it gave Alex a chance to meet individuals going through a similar experience; provided an opportunity for Alex to address her social anxiety (e.g., exposure to her feared stimulus); and offered a safe place for Alex to experiment with social transitioning.

Finally, Alex was referred to meet with a pediatric endocrinologist who specializes in transgender youth to discuss the protocols for and use of testosterone treatment for this patient population. This endocrinologist was consulted prior to Alex's appointment, and the comprehensive psychological/gender report was provided to offer recommendations and highlight the complexities of the case. Although testosterone was not recommended at the time of the evaluation, it was made clear to Alex that this would likely be an appropriate intervention in the future; thus, meeting with an endocrinologist would be worthwhile. Alex was enthusiastic about this recommendation, as it relayed the message to her that things were likely moving forward in her desired direction. Alex's parents were comfortable with this plan because they saw it as an opportunity to ask questions about the risks and benefits of using testosterone with a knowledgeable medical provider. This referral was also made because Alex was experiencing dysphoria related to menstruation. Therefore, the psychological evaluation report suggested that Alex be prescribed medication to stop menstruation, either with puberty-blocking medication or birth control (e.g., Depo-Provera). Alex was thrilled with this plan, and her parents were comfortable with this as well.

Case Discussion

This case provides an example of the complexity that can accompany transgender youth seeking medical interventions. Although many transgender individuals seeking medical interventions experience co-occurring mental health concerns, these are often determined to be secondary to the gender identity issue. This applies to adolescents as well; however, these transgender patients carry the added complexity of adolescent development, which includes cognitive, emotional, physical, and developmental factors. Adolescent development is complex for all youth, cisgender and transgender, and for this reason, applying a developmentally informed consent process is critical. This process often includes a comprehensive evaluation that is both affirming of a youth's gender identity yet takes into account many aspects of their development in order to contextualize their assertion and desired intervention.

This case illustrates how we might approach each of the questions posed at the beginning of the chapter. Following is a discussion of each.

1. For adolescent gender diverse patients presenting with significant anxiety and requesting hormone treatment, how well controlled should the anxiety be prior to the individual starting medical treatment for the gender dysphoria?

   In Alex's case, it was unclear how much the gender dysphoria was the primary cause of her anxiety and how much her gender dysphoria simply exacerbated it. Given the positive psychiatric history and the duration of Alex's anxiety symptoms (since childhood), it was hypothesized that the anxiety would have likely been present with or without the gender dysphoria. It is unrealistic to expect transgender individuals to experience no anxiety or have it significantly reduced prior to socially and physically transitioning; thus, it would not be recommended that the absence of anxiety symptoms be a requirement prior to considering medical intervention. However, in Alex's particular case, it did seem appropriate to recommend treatment for her anxiety while simultaneously providing supportive therapy to assist her with taking social transition steps. Doing this allowed Alex to begin to address her anxiety symptoms while simultaneously moving forward with her transition in a way that felt safe, supported, and manageable.
2. How important is it for adolescent gender diverse patients to explore the ways in which their anxiety may and may not be related to their gender dysphoria, and how much of this exploration should occur prior to the youth starting hormonal intervention?

   Similar to the response to the question above, it may not always be necessary for transgender individuals to explore their mental health symptoms at length prior to starting a medical intervention to address their gender dysphoria. Requiring this may inadvertently relay the message that their gender dysphoria may be a result of a mental health disorder and that by addressing the mental health symptoms, the gender dysphoria may improve. There is no research to support this conceptualization of gender dysphoria and approaching patients' narratives this way is pathologizing.

In Alex's case, her parents questioned whether she was identifying as transgender because of her difficulty socially fitting in with her peers. In this way, one may wonder if Alex's anxiety is somehow leading her to seek an identity within a group that is accepting of her, and thereby decreasing her anxiety. The potential relationship between Alex's anxiety and her transgender identity may be worth exploring further in therapy; however, it may not be something that necessarily needs to be deeply understood prior to beginning social and/or physical transitions.

3. Is it reasonable to expect adolescent gender diverse patients to undergo some degree of social transition prior to the initiation of irreversible medical interventions?

   This question is difficult, particularly when considering the movement away from this requirement for transgender adults. Some transgender youth, their parents, and providers may feel that transgender adolescents should be approached the same way as transgender adults in terms of protocols used for starting medical interventions. However, due to the added complexity that adolescence brings, it is recommended that transgender adolescents be approached on an individual basis in this regard, paying particular attention to developmental issues [6].

   Alex's case was a perfect example of the complexities that can accompany transgender adolescents. In this case, Alex's complexities prevented her from feeling comfortable socially transitioning. A medical transition would have likely brought on changes that would have forced a social transition because secondary sex characteristics would have occurred (e.g., voice deepening, increased body hair), possibly making it difficult for Alex to manage the reality that stigma exists toward individuals who change their gender. For the reasons described previously, it was recommended that Alex experience some degree of social transition prior to starting irreversible medical interventions. It was made clear to Alex, however, that this recommendation was not made as a roadblock, but as a standard of care that was believed to be in her best interest, as it was perceived as a helpful step toward preventing harm to Alex. She was also encouraged to meet with a pediatric endocrinologist to discuss protocols used for testosterone treatment in transgender youth so that she could move forward in her decision-making process about this possible intervention. It was clear when meeting with Alex that she did not have much knowledge about the effects of testosterone, and she was indifferent about some of the effects that were likely to occur. It was also recommended that Alex talk with the endocrinologist about medication to stop menstruation, as this seemed to be an intervention that would provide some relief and has no long-term, irreversible effects.

4. How important is it for time to be spent with parents of gender diverse patients to hear and validate their concerns and provide education and support prior to the adolescent beginning medical interventions?

   In almost all cases, including Alex's, it is critical for the parents of transgender youth to have the opportunity to share their story and their concerns with a mental health provider who is able to express empathy for their experience. Parents may feel silenced by affirming providers whose main focus is supporting the transgender youth. As the caregivers who have known their children the longest and most intimately, neglecting to hear their story leaves out a critical component of the transgender youth's picture. Additionally, transgender youth do best when they have the support of their parents, but parents are often unable to provide optimal support if they have not had the opportunity to feel heard and validated. The loss and grief that many parents of transgender youth experience can make it nearly impossible for them to support their child at times. Due to the stage of emotional development many adolescents are in, it is often difficult for them to appreciate the reasons for and depth of their parents' concerns. Working with a skilled therapist, both trained in adolescent development and family work, and knowledgeable about the unique needs of transgender adolescents and their families, is the ideal treatment for cases like Alex's.

Conclusion

In summary, transgender adolescents are an incredibly courageous and complicated patient population with whom more and more providers are given the opportunity to work. Having worked with hundreds of these youth and families, I can safely say that I have yet to approach a situation that is not both rewarding and uniquely challenging. Alex's case illustrates how anxiety, coupled with a later identification as transgender, can be clinically complex. Although an individualized approached is strongly recommended when working with transgender youth, applying some of the principles described in this chapter will likely help guide treatment for similarly presenting youth.

References

1. Spack NP, Edwards-Leeper L, Feldman HA, Leibowitz S, Mandel F, Diamond DA, et al. Children and adolescents with gender identity disorder referred to a pediatric medical center. Pediatrics. 2012;129(3):418–25.
2. Reisner SL, Vetters RV, Leclerc M, Zaslow S, Wolfrum S, Shumer D, et al. Mental health of transgender youth in care at an adolescent urban community health center: a matched retrospective cohort study. J Adolesc Health. 2016;56:274–9.
3. Edwards-Leeper L, Feldman A, Henry R, Lash B, Shumer D, Tishelman A. Psychological profile of the first sample of transgender youth presenting for medical intervention in a U.S. Pediatric Gender Center. Psychol Sex Orientat Gend Divers. 2017;4(3):374–82.
4. de Vries ALC, McGuire JK, Steensma TD, Wagenaar ECF, Doreleijers AH, Cohen-Kettenis PT. Young adult psychological outcome after puberty suppression and gender reassignment. Pediatrics. 2014;134:2013–958. https://doi.org/10.1542/peds.2013-2958.
5. Edwards-Leeper L, Spack NP. Psychological evaluation and medical treatment of transgender youth in an interdisciplinary "Gender Management Service" (GeMS) in a major pediatric center. J Homosex. 2012;59(3):321–36.

6. Edwards-Leeper L, Leibowitz S, Sangganjanavanich VF. Affirmative practice with transgender and gender non-conforming youth: expanding the model. Psychol Sex Orientat Gend Divers. 2016;3(2):165–72.
7. Ryan C, Russell ST, Huebner D, Diaz R, Sanchez J. Family acceptance in adolescence and the health of LGBT young adults. J Child Adolesc Psychiatr Nurs. 2010;23(4):205–13.
8. Olson KR, Durwood L, DeMeules M, McLaughlin KA. Mental health of transgender children who are supported in their identities. Pediatrics. 2015;137(3):2015–3223. https://doi.org/10.1542/peds.2015-3223.

Chapter 10
Trauma Stabilization and Recovery in a Transgender Latina: A Retrospective Case Example

Marco A. Hidalgo

Introduction

In comparison with children who conform to gender role expectations, gender-nonconforming children (regardless of their gender identity) are at greater risk of experiencing ridicule, discrimination, or victimization from family or peers, and these stressors have been found to increase their vulnerability to develop psychiatric conditions in adolescence including depression, anxiety, posttraumatic stress disorder (PTSD), and suicidality [1–5]. Gender-nonconforming and transgender youth exhibit higher rates of psychiatric problems than both youth without gender nonconformity [6] and cisgender, heterosexual youth [7]. The development of certain psychiatric conditions in adolescence has been tied to negative childhood experiences, including family rejection [8]. Minority stress theory postulates that sexual and gender minorities (e.g., lesbian, gay, bisexual, transgender (LGBT) individuals) may be especially susceptible to negative mental, physical, and behavioral health outcomes resulting from direct victimization and institutional forms of social discrimination on account of their sexual identity and/or gender identity/expression [9, 10].

Experiences of childhood sexual abuse are traumatic events that may also precipitate a host of negative mental health outcomes in heterosexual as well as LGBT populations [1, 3, 11–13]. Childhood sexual abuse is considered any form of sexual contact between a child and a person at least 5 years older and may consist of genital touching or fondling and vaginal, anal, or oral intercourse (or attempted intercourse) [14]. According to one meta-analysis of studies conducted among presumably cis-

M. A. Hidalgo, PhD
Division of Adolescent and Young Adult Medicine, Center for Transyouth Health and Development, Children's Hospital Los Angeles, Keck School of Medicine of the University of Southern California, Los Angeles, CA, USA
e-mail: mahidalgo@chla.usc.edu

A. Janssen, S. Leibowitz (eds.), *Affirmative Mental Health Care for Transgender and Gender Diverse Youth*, https://doi.org/10.1007/978-3-319-78307-9_10

gender samples (i.e., demographic data on sex assigned at birth and gender identity not reported), childhood sexual abuse was associated with increased lifetime diagnosis of psychiatric problems such as depression, anxiety, PTSD, as well as suicide attempts [15]. Those with histories of childhood sexual abuse are also more likely to be sexually revictimized later in life—1.8 times more likely in females and 5.5 times more likely in males [for a review, see 13]. No known research has examined revictimization in transgender people.

A retrospective study examined individuals assigned male sex at birth who had histories of childhood sexual abuse. Those with histories of childhood gender nonconformity were significantly more likely to have experienced PTSD, depression, and suicidality in adolescence and emerging adulthood than those without childhood gender nonconformity [5]. This finding was consistent with other research findings that childhood gender nonconformity may moderate the relationship between childhood sexual abuse and PTSD risk in adulthood [16]. Other recent studies of assigned males found an association between childhood gender nonconformity and childhood sexual abuse [5, 17]. It is conceivable that this association, in fact, suggests a unidirectional likelihood that gender-nonconforming individuals assigned male at birth are susceptible to sexual abuse on account of their gender expression. These associations do not likely suggest the opposite—that children exposed to sexual abuse are likely to then exhibit gender nonconformity—as there is a lack of evidence to suggest that childhood gender nonconformity "manifests" as a result of adverse childhood experiences including childhood sexual abuse [for a review, see 18]. Moreover, according to both professional consensus [19] and tenets of the gender affirmative model of multidisciplinary care among gender-diverse youth [20], variations in both gender identities and gender expression are considered aspects of human diversity and not inherently pathological in nature. According to these principles, multidisciplinary approaches to care should be individualized and comprehensive to ensure gender-diverse youth and their families receive medical and mental health treatment (when appropriate) in accordance with professional standards of care [21, 22].

Over the past two decades, the field of trauma psychology has become increasingly dedicated to examining resiliency, thereby exploring how, for some, experiences of adversity precipitate increases in personal wellness and advancement to levels that exceed pre-traumatic exposure. Specifically, the concept of *posttraumatic growth* is defined as a process (i.e., a non-static phenomenon) "of positive psychological change experienced as a result of the struggle with highly challenging life circumstances" [23]. Indicators of posttraumatic growth are personal and interpersonal and may include an increased sense of life appreciation, an increased sense of personal strength and recognition of new life possibilities, as well as healthier and more fulfilling intimate relationships [24]. Uniquely identified among survivors of childhood emotional, physical, or sexual abuse are additional mechanisms that yield growth including experiences of validation, nurturing, mastery, as well as an increased value for healthy relationships [25].

Case Report

The clinical material presented here consists of a case of brief (i.e., 15 sessions) trauma-informed psychotherapy focused on acute symptom stabilization and involving a 20-year-old, bicultural, transgender Latina (i.e., assigned male at birth) with a history of childhood sexual abuse. The material will be presented in three sequential sections that coincide with (1) assessment and treatment planning, (2) mid-treatment, and (3) termination/closure. This chapter will illustrate the patient's experiences of victimization related to her gender identity/expression, the negative psychosocial outcomes related to these experiences (including minority stress), and signs indicating a process of posttraumatic growth. To protect the confidentiality of this patient, all references to identifying information and dates have been changed or omitted.

The reader may have a priori questions and considerations when reviewing such a case, including:

- Can brief cognitive-behavioral approaches also be trauma-informed approaches?
- In what ways can gender-affirmative therapy also be trauma-informed?

These questions will be addressed through case material and, more explicitly, later in the chapter.

Diagnosis and Assessment

This writer had the pleasure of initially meeting "Cristal" one day in October, when she presented to a multidisciplinary gender development clinic with interest in initiating feminizing hormone therapy and to begin psychotherapy with this writer aimed at managing symptoms of anxiety and processing a "breakup." Cristal was female identified and assigned male at birth. She was sexually attracted to cisgender males and self-identified as "straight." She was a naturalized US citizen but born in a Latin American country. She was bicultural, reporting strong acculturative ties to both the USA and her Latin American country of origin (LAC). She was fluently bilingual in English and Spanish. Her parents divorced when she was 14 years old, and her father relocated to LAC. Cristal described a longstanding history of gender nonconformity extending from childhood through adolescence. She disclosed being transgender to her family at age 17 and described her father as more accepting than her mother.

One month prior to meeting this writer, Cristal returned to the USA from LAC, where she resided for the past 1.5 years, fully socially transitioned as female—first residing with her father and stepmother and then with friends. Ultimately, for her final 4 months in LAC, she resided with a 26-year-old cisgender male partner (Alejandro). Upon returning to the USA, Cristal reverted to living full time as male because she reported that her mother continued to be unsupportive and had explicitly forbidden Cristal from transitioning socially or medically. In fact, though Cristal was listed under her mother's health insurance plan, she requested that her services for these sessions be billed to her directly so as to conceal from her mother her involvement in gender-affirming services (fortunately, this writer was successful at gaining coverage for Cristal's session fees through a charitable hospital fund). Cristal did not complete high school, having left for LAC at the start of her senior year. She reported that she emigrated to LAC to escape her mother's ridicule regarding her gender identity. She was currently enrolled in classes to earn a general education diploma (GED) at a local community college. She planned to sit for her GED exam in 2–3 months. Cristal was seeking employment in order to save money to move on her own. Cristal reported looking forward to initiating hormone therapy because she believed she took "a big step back" after relocating to the USA and no longer living full time as female. Cristal also stated that her mother could eventually help subsidize Cristal's rent. Cristal was unsure if her mother would continue to support her financially (or with shelter), if Cristal initiated feminizing hormone therapy. Regarding finding alternative housing, Cristal stated that she could make such arrangements "next week, if I had to"; however, she was unclear as to where she would relocate.

Cristal's recent psychiatric history was significant for anxiety symptoms. She had returned to the USA due, in part, to the dissolution of her relationship and also due to challenges with managing anxiety symptoms consistent with PTSD. Crystal had a history of chronic PTSD having experienced these symptoms since mid-adolescence "but now they're just getting worse." The worsening of these symptoms appeared to result from exposure to traumatic violence beginning in May. These exposures included receiving ongoing verbal, emotional, and physical partner violence from Alejandro including an incident in May in which he choked her until she lost consciousness. A second traumatic exposure occurred in August. The incident involved a group of LAC male police officers verbally harassing her, arresting her, physically victimizing her, and threatening to kill her. Cristal described fearing for her life in both incidents. At this time, Cristal denied experiencing any earlier traumatic difficulties prior to these experiences.

Cristal's mood was negatively impacted by her symptoms of acute anxiety, gender dysphoria, and by factors related to her adjustment back to the USA. Primary stressors included her mourning the loss of Alejandro, whom she described as both "a total jerk" and "the only man who will ever love me for me," her belief that she regressed in terms of her gender transition after relocating to the USA, and her loss of a gender-affirming social network. Cristal regularly had hopeless thoughts such as "I'm going to end up dying alone and from AIDS" and "Guys will only want me for sex [and not a relationship]." Cristal denied any history of suicidal ideation or homicidal ideation. However, Cristal reported that since returning to the USA she had developed an increase in thoughts that she would passively succumb to death "by catching HIV and dying that way." She denied having undergone an HIV antibody test in the past year and feared that the results would indicate an HIV-positive serostatus.

Cristal described being a "smiley," "sensitive," "loving" child. She recalled "always knowing" she was female. She shared that, as a 5-year-old, she would often tuck her penis between her legs to resemble a vagina and attempt to cross-dress in her mother's clothes. As a child, she recalled being ridiculed by her father on account of her gender nonconformity. At age 12, she came out as "gay" in the hope that her parents would be more tolerant of her gender expression. Instead, she recalled her parents reacting negatively and taking her to Evangelical Christian services where she was often berated by pastors and fellow churchgoers. Cristal recalled her mother regularly telling her she would "live a hard life" and that gay people acquire and transmit AIDS. She also recalled that around this time her parents began regularly taking her to receive "hormone medication" which she later discovered to be testosterone injections "because they wanted to make me more manly." Cristal received this treatment for at least 6–8 months. She recalled experiencing anatomic dysphoria prior to this period and, with this treatment, came more rapid virilization and the development of unwanted secondary sex characteristics (e.g., voice deepening, facial hair growth, muscular frame) that exacerbated her body dissatisfaction.

Cristal denied any significant medical history. Cristal also denied any previous psychiatric hospitalization or psychotherapy; however, just shortly before she relocated from LAC to the USA, she filled a prescription of sertraline (i.e., Zoloft) from a primary care physician to manage panic symptoms (without agoraphobia) but had not taken the medication for fear of weight gain.

In terms of risk behavior, Cristal endorsed a history of sex work spanning 4–6 months, which concluded in August, before she departed LAC—"I stopped because it just wasn't for me." She denied any history of sexual assault. In addition to HIV testing, she had not undergone testing for sexually transmitted infections/diseases (STI) in nearly 1 year. Cristal's substance use history was significant for minimal cannabis use several years prior, and she reported "experimenting" with crystal meth on two occasions while dating Alejandro.

Based on the clinical assessment data collected and presented above, this writer assigned Cristal the following psychiatric diagnoses after providing her with education about each condition, its prognosis, and method of treatment. She reported that each diagnosis accurately reflected the affective, cognitive, and behavioral challenges she was managing. For a description of each diagnosis, please refer to the *Diagnostic and Statistical Manual of Mental Disorders, Fifth Edition* (DSM-5) [26].

- Gender dysphoria in adulthood
- Posttraumatic stress disorder
- Adjustment disorder with depressed mood
- V15.41: Personal history of spouse or partner violence, physical

Management

Cristal articulated a strong desire that treatment focus on addressing her acute anxiety symptoms and adjustment concerns. She also stated that, due to her pursuit of employment and alternative housing, she was unaware of how long she could engage in psychotherapy. She was very enthusiastic about this writer's recommendation that for the first 4 weeks, she receive a concentrated dose (i.e., 60-min sessions twice per week) of cognitive behavioral therapy (CBT) aimed at stabilizing trauma symptoms. To orient Cristal to the process of trauma recovery, this writer described Herman's developmental stage model of recovery from chronic and complex PTSD—safety/stabilization, remembrance/mourning, and reconnection [12]. This writer and Cristal then discussed how her desire to focus on acute symptom management fell nicely within the model's first stage, "safety/stabilization." This writer discussed with Cristal that, should she choose in the future, the treatment plan could be revised to address additional trauma recovery stages. Given Cristal's report of trauma-like symptoms since mid-adolescence, this writer also considered it possible that Cristal may disclose a childhood trauma history after building greater rapport with this writer. Cognitive processing therapy is a trauma-informed CBT considered a "gold standard" treatment for trauma symptoms resulting from interpersonal forms of violence including physical and sexual assault and childhood abuse [27, 28]. This writer also selected this approach as it is intended to be a short-term treatment, with 8–12 1-hour-long sessions serving as a general guideline for care [29].

In addition to CBT, individual supportive therapy focused on facilitating grief processes related to romantic relationship dissolution. Adjunctively, this writer referred Cristal to several gender-affirming support groups that were free and led by LGBT-affiliated organizations.

Cristal declined this writer's recommendation to seek an evaluation for psychopharmacological intervention after expressing concerns for weight gain and "not wanting to depend on drugs to get better." This writer also initially recommended that Cristal consider inviting her mother to future sessions to either discuss gender development or Cristal's gender transition; however, Cristal declined after citing that her mother was not yet open to understanding her and that this involvement would threaten the stability of her housing. To help address gender dysphoria, this writer also recommended that Cristal continue her assessment of readiness regarding initiating feminizing hormone therapy. This writer discussed the possibility that Cristal's initiating hormone therapy would potentially complicate matters at home and potentially lead to her mother asking her to move out. Cristal maintained confidence that she would find alternative housing if such concerns arose. Last, this writer recommended community-based drop-in groups: one group, for transgender youth aged 18 and up, which she attended regularly, and a second group for LGBT survivors of relationship violence, which she ultimately attended three to four times due to conflicts in her work schedule.

Mid-Treatment (Sessions 4–12)

Per her treatment plan, Cristal attended all eight sessions scheduled on a twice-per-week basis. She had acquired employment as a janitor and began saving money to rent a room. She worked overnight shifts where she was known by the name assigned to her at birth "because people wouldn't really accept me there." Her motivation toward treatment did not waiver during this period. On several occasions she attended therapy sessions at 7:00 a.m., following the end of her overnight shift.

Regarding trauma symptoms, she responded well to cognitive processing therapy, including imaginal exposure-based tasks that involved her managing anxiety symptoms that surfaced while recalling aspects of recent traumatic incidents. Per Cristal's request, these sessions also incorporated discussions of Alejandro's treatment of her. We would reference the "LGBT power and control wheel" [30], which highlights various behaviors that constitute partner violence (e.g., intimidation, emotional abuse, economic abuse, etc.), and concepts of Walker's three-stage model (tension-building, acute incident, honeymoon phase) referred to as the *cycle of violence* [for a full description, see 31]. Time was also devoted to identifying aspects of healthful relationships. During this period, Cristal shifted in her characterization of Alejandro's behavior—from "he was just possessive" and "passionate" to "abusive" and "just not something you do to someone you love." She began to share her fantasies for an ideal relationship—mutual respect, tenderness, and unconditional acceptance.

By her eighth session, symptoms of anxiety began to stabilize and decrease, and Cristal reported feeling "calmer than I ever have." She believed that the adaptive coping skills (relaxation skills, cognitive restructuring skills, etc.) and self-empathy she was learning were forms of self-nurturance. In one of these discussions 3 weeks into treatment, she went on to state that the only resemblance of childhood nurturance she received was from an older male relative (10 years her senior). She went on to state that from ages 5–11 years, this male relative sexually abused her. Cristal reported feeling immensely guilty about these encounters because she perceived having initiated some of them over the years. Over time, her abuser would threaten to disclose to Cristal's parents that she had initiated the encounters, which frightened Cristal into silence. She reported not having disclosed this history to anyone prior to this writer.

This writer and Cristal revisited the treatment plan to determine how much it should incorporate this childhood history of sexual abuse. Cristal stated that she was not comfortable discussing the details of this history at this time but was most interested in exploring its impact on her life now. In these early discussions, she recognized parallels between her histories of sexual abuse and intimate partner violence (IPV)—"It was that same cycle of violence—being real nice to me in order to get what they wanted, then treating me bad again."

During this time, Cristal was reporting a greater frequency of sex partners whom she had met online and a tendency to acquiesce with their requests to engage in condomless receptive anal sex. Her sexual risk behavior she tied to a cognitive distortion in the form of HIV-related fatalistic thinking (e.g., "it's only a matter of time that I get HIV," "I'm surprised I don't have [HIV] yet"). This writer educated Cristal on minority stress, and she shared examples from her past that reflected these experiences (e.g., ridicule from father, receiving testosterone treatment, negative statements regarding LGBT people). She also identified that she had internalized distorted messages from her mother regarding an inevitability of acquiring HIV/AIDS. Identifying possible sources of this negativistic thinking appeared to motivate Cristal toward behavior change, and she began to identify effective replacement thoughts rooted in self-efficacy (e.g., "I can protect myself." "A sexy girl is an assertive one."). She also agreed to undergo HIV and STI testing, and all results were negative. To help assuage her challenges with consistent condom use, this writer also referred Cristal for consultation for HIV-related pre-exposure prophylaxis (PrEP), a once-a-day pill that has been found to be effective in preventing HIV infection in transgender women who have sex with men [32, 33]. By the end of mid-therapy, Cristal had received a prescription for PrEP and reported taking the pill daily although she was less sexually active than in previous weeks.

Termination/Closure (Sessions 14–18)

Cristal's last several sessions inadvertently occurred every other week or sometimes with 3 weeks passing between visits. She reported being very busy, and relying solely on public transportation to travel great lengths to school and work, she also had limited time. While continuing to work and attend GED courses, she had also moved into her own room in the two-bedroom apartment belonging to a new friend—a transgender Latina 3 years her senior—whom she had befriended at a social support group. Cristal had recently begun blogging short videos about her transition and received many positive comments and feedback from the hundreds of transgender women who had begun to follow her page. Her roommate, a more successful and seasoned blogger, had promoted Cristal's page, which increased Cristal's number of followers tenfold. She was very proud of her success. She reported feeling a great sense of comfort in her body and presented more often as her affirmed gender in most settings (except work). She also reported that her mother appeared to be more tolerable of Cristal that she had referred to Cristal as her "daughter" on several occasions and also offered to help her either subsidize her rent or estrogen therapy—"I can't believe it!"

Cristal began drawing links between her abuse history, a growing recognition of internalized transphobia, and core beliefs that she was "not worthy" of receiving love from others. She actively identified how this belief might have contributed to her tendency to self-deprecate and place the desires of sexual partners before her own safer-sex intentions. A growing knowledge of what constituted partner abuse allowed her to challenge self-beliefs that she was responsible for the abuse she received from Alejandro. However, she found it difficult to displace self-blame when considering experiences of childhood sexual abuse. This difficulty stemmed from a belief that she was to blame for her abuse since there were times in which she perceived having initiated the encounters and sometimes enjoyed them. Cristal eventually began to shed this responsibility when she disputed it with observations from her childhood sociocultural environment, where needs of children were not prioritized by adults; therefore, "even if I did want something, he should've said 'no' because [in my family] grown-ups had no problem saying 'no' to us kids."

After a series of no-call, no-show appointments, this writer received a phone message from Cristal in which she requested to speak by phone regarding her interest in continuing therapy. When this writer spoke with her, she shared that she "has never felt better" and felt confident in her ability to continue managing anxiety symptoms based on what she had learned in therapy thus far, and "maybe I can come in and visit you one day soon?" This writer agreed and congratulated Cristal on the successes she accomplished in therapy. They reviewed areas of continued growth, including doing her best to cultivate healthful platonic and romantic/sexual relationships.

Clinical Pearls/Pitfalls

This case material illustrated themes from scientific literature pertaining to the negative outcomes (aside from suicidality) associated with both childhood sexual abuse and gender nonconformity in individuals assigned male at birth. However, aside from presenting a clinical dimension to these deficit-focused themes, the case also highlighted aspects of resilience present in this young transgender Latina.

For example, perhaps even at the start of therapy, Cristal appeared to be on a process toward posttraumatic growth as she was motivated toward achieving self-understanding, positive behavior change, and psychosocial wellness that exceeded her pre-trauma levels. Over the course of treatment, Cristal became aware of long-standing negative patterns tied to core beliefs. She examined ways in which her negative core beliefs (e.g., "I'm not worthy") influenced her tendency to self-deprecate, engage in risky sexual behavior, and contribute to negativistic thinking patterns. Cristal also developed a keen awareness regarding patterns of partner abuse in her relationship, which she previously had not recognized as dysfunctional and counter to her ideals in a romantic relationship. This awareness allowed her to challenge self-beliefs that she was responsible for the abuse she received from her ex-boyfriend, and she also eventually drew parallels between patterns of childhood sexual abuse and intimate partner violence.

To this writer, perhaps Cristal's improved sense of creativity and increased effort to maintain gender-affirming social support were most obvious signs of posttraumatic growth. She accomplished this through tireless efforts at reconnecting with community via social support groups and eventually through her video blogging. These connections, in turn, appeared to bring a multitude of personal resources—greater self-esteem, friendships, and a safe place to live.

Several a priori questions were posed earlier in this chapter. From the case described here, it is hopefully clear for the reader that, indeed, brief CBT approaches can also be trauma-informed. Psychotherapies that are CBT-oriented, in particular, can very easily translate to trauma-informed work. Fundamentally, they are guided by a "collaborative empiricism," an approach in which decision-making about treatment priorities and pacing reside with both the patient and the provider. CBT approaches also include many very effective and brief psychotherapeutic techniques that, when learned, can increase a patient's repertoire of adaptive skills.

Gender-affirmative therapy can also be trauma-informed. In this case, this writer demonstrated a gender-affirmative orientation by being informed about gender development, trans Latina culture, and validating the patient's affirmed identity from the start of treatment. Being gender affirming can also include discussing "readiness" for hormone therapy in a way that encourages them to consider its interplay with environmental stressors, which should not be confused with discouraging a patient from engaging in this medically necessary treatment because of deficits in their psychosocial support system. For example, this writer assured the patient that she was "ready" to begin hormone therapy whenever she chose, and he also appropriately expressed his concerns to Cristal that the timing of hormone therapy could jeopardize her somewhat precarious housing with her mother. Expressing this concern allowed for both the patient and this writer to problem-solve so that the patient had a plan to manage these potential stressors once initiating hormone therapy.

Perhaps, most importantly, a clinician delivering trauma-focused treatment to a gender-nonconforming/transgender child, adolescent, or young adult should follow a developmentally informed trauma recovery model such as Herman's [for a full description, see 12]. Reliance on such a model may engender further safety and stabilization for the patient as the model provides them with a helpful frame and sequence of staging in which trauma recovery occurs. This may also allow for the patient to choose, as Cristal did here, how, to what degree, and when to address trauma recovery.

Conclusion

This case illustrated experiences of childhood victimization in a transgender Latina (i.e., assigned male at birth) that were associated with her childhood history of gender nonconformity. Also illustrated by this case were negative psychosocial outcomes that appeared to be associated with these experiences. While the brief therapy employed a cognitive behavioral approach that addressed acute symptoms of a more recent traumatic event, the patient appeared to also apply these new cognitive frameworks to understand her past experiences of trauma. She also began to consider the potential impact of these past experiences on her psychosocial well-being. A brief discussion highlighted ways in which this patient exhibited posttraumatic growth.

References

1. D'Augelli AR, Grossman AH, Starks MT. Childhood gender atypicality, victimization, and PTSD among lesbian, gay, and bisexual youth. J Interpers Violence. 2006;21(11):1462–82.
2. Garofalo R, Deleon J, Osmer E, Doll M, Harper GW. Overlooked, misunderstood and at-risk: exploring the lives and HIV risk of ethnic minority male-to-female transgender youth. J Adolesc Health. 2006;38(3):230–6.

3. Roberts AL, Rosario M, Corliss HL, Koenen KC, Bryn Austin S. Elevated risk of posttraumatic stress in sexual minority youths: mediation by childhood abuse and gender nonconformity. Am J Public Health. 2012;102(8):1587–93.
4. Skidmore W, Linsenmeier J, Bailey J. Gender nonconformity and psychological distress in lesbians and gay men. Arch Sex Behav. 2006;35(6):685–97.
5. Hidalgo MA, Kuhns LM, Kwon S, Mustanski B, Garofalo R. The impact of childhood gender expression on childhood sexual abuse and psychopathology among young men who have sex with men. Child Abuse Negl. 2015;46:103–12.
6. Reisner SL, Vetters R, Leclerc M, Zaslow S, Wolfrum S, Shumer D, et al. Mental health of transgender youth in care at an adolescent urban community health center: a matched retrospective cohort study. J Adolesc Health. 2015;56(3):274–9.
7. Mustanski BS, Garofalo R, Emerson EM. Mental health disorders, psychological distress, and suicidality in a diverse sample of lesbian, gay, bisexual, and transgender youths. Am J Public Health. 2010;100(12):2426–32.
8. Ryan C, Russell ST, Huebner D, Diaz RM, Sanchez J. Family acceptance in adolescence and the health of LGBT young adults. J Child Adolesc Psychiatr Nurs. 2010;23(4):205–13.
9. Meyer IH. Minority stress and mental health in gay men. J Health Soc Behav. 1995;36:38–56.
10. Testa RJ, Habarth J, Peta J, Balsam K, Bockting W. Development of the gender minority stress and resilience measure. Psychol Sex Orient Gend Divers. 2014;2(1):65–77.
11. Benoit E, Downing MJ. Childhood sexual experiences among substance-using non-gay identified Black men who have sex with men and women. Child Abuse Negl. 2013;37:679–90.
12. Herman JL. Trauma and recovery. New York, NY: Basic Books; 1997.
13. Classen CC, Palesh OG, Aggarwal R. Sexual revictimization: a review of the empirical literature. Trauma Violence Abuse. 2005;6(2):103–29.
14. Andrews G, Corry J, Slade T, Issakidis C, Swanston H. Child sexual abuse. In: Ezzati M, Lopez AD, Rodgers A, Murray CJL, editors. Comparative quantification of health risks: global and regional burden of disease attributable to selected major risk factors. Geneva: World Health Organization; 2004. p. 1851–940.
15. Chen LP, Murad MH, Paras ML, Colbenson KM, Sattler AL, Goranson EN, et al., editors. Sexual abuse and lifetime diagnosis of psychiatric disorders: systematic review and meta-analysis. Mayo Clin Proc. 2010;85(7):618–29.
16. Roberts AL, Rosario M, Corliss HL, Koenen KC, Bryn Austin S. Childhood gender nonconformity: a risk indicator for childhood abuse and posttraumatic stress in youth. Pediatrics. 2012;129:410–7.
17. Bandini E, Fisher AD, Ricca V, Ristori J, Meriggiola MC, Jannini EA, et al. Childhood maltreatment in subjects with male-to-female gender identity disorder. Int J Impot Res. 2011;23:276–85.
18. Sánchez FJ, Vilain E. Transgender identities: research and controversies. In: Patterson CJ, D'Augelli AR, editors. Handbook of psychology and sexual orientation. New York, NY: Oxford University Press; 2013.
19. SAMHSA. Ending conversion therapy: supporting and affirming LGBTQ youth. Substance Abuse and Mental Health Services Administration, HHS Publication No. (SMA) 15-4928, 2015.
20. Hidalgo MA, Ehrensaft D, Tishelman AC, Clark LF, Garofalo R, Rosenthal SM, et al. The gender affirmative model: what we know and what we aim to learn. Hum Dev. 2013;56(5):285–90.
21. Hembree WC, Cohen-Kettenis P, Delemarre-van de Waal HA, Gooren LJ, Meyer WJ, Spack NP, et al. Endocrine treatment of transsexual persons: an Endocrine Society clinical practice guideline. J Clin Endocrinol Metab. 2009;94(9):3132–54.
22. Coleman E, Bockting W, Botzer M, Cohen-Kettenis P, DeCuypere G, Feldman J, et al. Standards of care for the health of transsexual, transgender, and gender-nonconforming people, version 7. Int J Transgenderism. 2012;13(4):165–232.
23. Tedeschi RG, Calhoun LG. Posttraumatic growth: conceptual foundations and empirical evidence. Psychol Inquiry. 2004;15(1):1–18.
24. Tedeschi RG, Calhoun LG. The posttraumatic growth inventory: measuring the positive legacy of trauma. J Traumatic Stress. 1996;9:455–72.

25. Woodward C, Joseph S. Postive change processes and post-traumatic growth in people who have experience childhood abuse: understanding vehicles of change. Psychol Psychother Theory Res Pract. 2003;76:267–83.
26. APA. Diagnostic and statistical manual of mental disorders—fifth edition (DSM-5)™. Arlington, VA: American Psychiatric Association; 2013.
27. Cahill SP, Rothbaum BO, Resick PA, Follette VM. Cognitive-behavioral therapy for adults. In: Foa EB, Keane TM, Friedman MJ, Cohen JA, editors. Effective treatments for PTSD: practice guidelines from the International Society for Traumatic Stress Studies. New York, NY: Guilford Press; 2008. p. 139–222.
28. Kaysen D, Lostutter TW, Goines MA. Cognitive processing therapy for acute stress disorder resulting from an anti-gay assault. Cogn Behav Pract. 2005;12(3):278–89.
29. Foa EB, Keane TM, Friedman MJ, Cohen JA. Effective treatments for PTSD: practice guidelines from the International Society for Traumatic Stress Studies. New York, NY: Guilford Press; 2008.
30. Roe & Jagodinsky. Gay, lesbian, bisexual and trans power and control wheel. Austin, TX: Texas Council of Family Violence; n.d.
31. Walker LE. Psychology and domestic violence around the world. Am Psychol. 1999;54(1):21–9.
32. Grant RM, Anderson PL, McMahan V, Liu A, Amico KR, Mehrotra M, et al. Uptake of pre-exposure prophylaxis, sexual practices, and HIV incidence in men and transgender women who have sex with men: a cohort study. Lancet. 2014;14(9):820–9.
33. Veloso VG, Mesquita F, Grinszten B. Pre-exposure prophylaxis for men and transgender women who have sex with men in Brazil: opportunities and challenges. J Int AIDS Soc. 2015;18(4 Suppl 3):20010.

Chapter 11
Depression and Gender Dysphoria

Eric N. Boyum and Peter Daniolos

Introduction

Although transgender adolescents often experience angst related to the dissonance between experienced and assigned gender, most such youth with access to affirming care and supportive families will successfully navigate the transition from assigned/natal gender to experienced gender, growing into well-adjusted adults [1–3]. However, a significant minority will have one or more diagnosable mental health disorder, of which mood and anxiety disorders are among the most common. Depression among transgender youth can occur up to two to three times as often as among their cisgender peers, in contrast to more uncommon conditions like bipolar disorder and schizophrenia which have been observed at expected rates [4].

Since not all youth volunteer descriptions of their mood state, all transgender youth should be thoroughly assessed for depression. When depressed feelings emerge as an area of concern for a transgender youth, further evaluation should seek to understand what underlies their depressed state—for example, endogenous major depressive disorder, adjustment to external stressors, and/or anxiety related to incongruence between gender identity and pubertal changes. This chapter will present three cases of transgender adolescents, each with some degree of depressive distress. The underpinnings of each adolescent's dysphoria are discussed, culminating in formulations and rationale for therapeutic interventions.

E. N. Boyum, MD (✉) • P. Daniolos, MD
Department of Child and Adolescent Psychiatry, University of Iowa Stead Family Children's Hospital, Iowa City, IA, USA
e-mail: eboyum@mahaskahealth.org; peter-daniolos@uiowa.edu

A. Janssen, S. Leibowitz (eds.), *Affirmative Mental Health Care for Transgender and Gender Diverse Youth*, https://doi.org/10.1007/978-3-319-78307-9_11

Gender dysphoria and depression can predispose an individual toward self-injurious behavior including non-suicidal self-injury and suicidal behavior, both of which are found at higher rates among transgender individuals than their cisgender peers [5, 6]. One study of the mental health of transgender youth found that over half had considered suicide, and nearly one in three had made a suicide attempt [7]. As suicide is the second leading cause of death among all children, adolescents, and young adults aged 10–34 in the United States [8], interventions for depression and self-injurious thoughts or behaviors in transgender youth can be lifesaving. The cases presented here had some degree of self-directed violence in addition to depressive distress.

Summary of Key Clinical Questions

1. To what degree are depressive disorders and self-directed violence co-occurring with gender dysphoria throughout the developmental process?
2. What is the current theoretical framework for understanding how depression arises in transgender youth?
3. Why should clinicians pay attention to the vital relationships between transgender youth and their families? What role does parental support play?
4. How does a clinician ultimately determine whether hormone treatment will resolve a youth's acute depression or whether depression should be first treated by other means before a referral is made?

Co-occurring Depression and Self-Directed Violence in Gender Dysphoric Youth

Depression is common among both cisgender and transgender youth. Around 2% of all school-age children and 20% of youth will experience an episode of major depression [9]. Spack et al. reported that among youth aged 4–20 presenting to their gender clinic, depression was the most common psychiatric diagnosis, with around 1 in 4 having been diagnosed with a depressive disorder prior to initial gender clinic evaluation, over one-third of youth having been prescribed psychotropic medication, and almost 1 in 10 having been previously psychiatrically hospitalized [10].

Investigators have sought to understand the mental health of gender-nonconforming children using both dimensional and categorical assessments of a wide range of symptoms. Both internalizing (e.g., depression and anxiety) and externalizing (e.g., hyperactivity, aggression) problems are prevalent among children referred for gender nonconformity. Zucker and colleagues have reported that parents describe more behavioral problems on the Child Behavior Checklist (CBCL) for both natal boys and girls referred for gender-nonconforming behavior, compared to their cisgender siblings [11]. Yunger et al. [12] conducted a survey of children in two cohorts, grades 3–4 and grades 5–7. The children in each cohort were asked standardized questions about gender typicality, gender contentedness, and felt pressure for gender conformity. The results of this survey indicated that the greater the degree of gender nonconformity, gender discontent, and felt pressure for gender conformity, the less psychologically well-adjusted the children were likely to be 1 year later. Those children experiencing pressure to conform to expected gender-based behaviors were significantly more likely to have internalizing symptoms. Wallien et al. [13] assessed 120 gender dysphoric children aged 4–11 for psychiatric disorders based on a structured DSM-based parent interview. The results indicated that these children had a great deal of psychiatric comorbidity; 52% met criteria for at least one other psychiatric diagnosis. These children were most likely to have an anxiety disorder (over 30%), and mood disorders were found in 6% of the sample. Over the course of childhood development, some data indicate that gender-nonconforming children develop further emotional and behavioral problems as they get older. Zucker's group analyzed CBCL data from their Toronto-based gender clinic and found that the percentage of gender-nonconforming children within the clinical range on the CBCL increased in a linear fashion for each age cohort from ages 4–5 to ages 10–12 [14].

Transgender youth face additional challenges during the teenage years. De Ceglie et al. [15] described a number of demographic and clinical features of children and teens referred to their large European gender identity service. Teens (over 12 years of age) struggled with several clinical features related to mood disorders, though mood disorders themselves were not measured. Depression and "misery" were common in teenagers, doubling from 26% in the under 12 age group to 52% in the 12+ age group. Associated features of self-deprecation (33%), irritability (23%), and mood swings (22%) were common, and 75% reported relationship issues with their parents. De Vries et al. [1] found that, when using a structured diagnostic interview, the rate of depressive disorders in transgender teenagers age 10.5–18 was 12.4%, double the rate found by the same group in younger transgender children. Another group reported Beck Depression Inventory (BDI-II) scores for 101 trans youth aged 12–24 when entering their gender clinic, finding that 35% had clinically significant depressive symptoms and 11% had severe depressive symptoms [7].

In the teenage years, gender dysphoric youth may become eligible for puberty suppressing medical treatments to prevent further development of unwanted secondary sex characteristics and potentially will start cross-sex hormones and/or gender-affirming surgical interventions several years later to promote development of secondary sex characteristics of their experienced gender. While the above studies largely included only youth with limited experience with such interventions, de Vries et al. conducted a longitudinal study of psychological functioning of 55 gender dysphoric youth before medical intervention, after pubertal blockade, and after gender-affirming hormonal and surgical interventions [3]. In this sample, the mean BDI-II score at the initial assessment was quite low compared to those reported elsewhere for adolescents and did not improve with medical interventions; however, several other measures of psychological functioning improved with subsequent gender-affirming interventions—to the point that postoperative subjects had levels of psychological functioning within the normative range of their cisgender peers [3]. This is congruent with other longitudinal studies, which demonstrate similar improvements in psychological functioning after the provision of gender-affirming medical interventions (reviewed in Dhejne et al. [4]). Gender-affirming medical intervention clearly reduces the suffering of gender dysphoric adolescents when it is available and acceptable to the youth and their legal guardians. However, one cannot always rely on affirming medical interventions to resolve all torment among transgender youth.

Unfortunately, some depressed transgender adolescents and young adults will be injured or die as a result of self-directed violence. For decades, transgender youth have been included with sexual minorities, such as gay, lesbian, and bisexual youth, when rates of suicide have been discussed. Perhaps the first national attention given to the problem of suicide among LGBT youth was the 1989 Report of the Secretary's Task Force on Youth Suicide, which estimated that sexual minority youth comprised up to 30% of completed suicides among young people annually at that time [16]. Large national youth surveys have not included questions meant to identify transgender youth, thus limiting large-scale estimates of self-directed violence among transgender youth, with prevalence estimates for self-directed violence relying on smaller samples. Many studies have assessed rates of self-directed violence among LGBT youth as a whole, and subgroup analysis suggests that transgender youth have similar elevated rates of non-suicidal self-injury and suicide (see [17]). Many clinician researchers have commented on the high rates of suicidal ideation, non-suicidal self-injurious behavior (NSSI), and suicide attempts among referred transgender youth (Table 11.1). In the UK, Holt et al. [18], Skagerberg et al. [19], and De Ceglie et al. [15] have stratified such results by age and found that self-injurious behavior and suicide attempts were rare prior to age 12; the majority of suicide

Table 11.1 Studies of self-directed violence among transgender youth

Study (location)	Age	Non-suicidal self-injury (%)	Suicidal ideation (%)	Suicide attempt (%)
Spack et al. [10] (Massachusetts, USA)	4–20	21	NR	9
De Ceglie et al. [15] (London, UK)	11 ± 4	18	NR	13
Olson et al. [7] (California, USA)	12–24	NR	51	30
Grossman and D'Augelli [5] (New York/Pennsylvania, USA)	14–21	NR	45	26
Skagerberg et al. [19] (London, UK)	12.6 ± 3.2	24	14	10
Reisner et al. [22] (Massachusetts, USA)	19.7 ± 3.1	17	31	17
Mustanski et al. [2] (Illinois, USA)	16–20	NR	10	10
Holt et al. [18] (London, UK)	5–17	39	35	13

NR not reported

attempts occurred between ages 12 and 15 in the Skagerberg study. While the rates of NSSI are not largely different from American and German rates of NSSI in the general population, the rates of suicide attempts are substantially larger in most of the samples [20]. Based upon parent-reported CBCL data, Zucker's Canadian group found a similar trend that both suicidal ideation and self-harm/suicide attempts increase with age [21].

Neither depression nor self-directed violence occurs in a vacuum. The recently reported GLSEN National School Climate Survey indicates that transgender youth were most likely of all LGBT youth to have negative experiences at school, and three quarters reported feeling unsafe at school because of their gender expression (p. 84) [23]. A growing body of evidence suggests that stigmatization [6, 24, 25], victimization [24–27], and rejection by peers and family [6, 26, 28, 29] all play important roles in the development of depression and self-directed violence in transgender youth. Some youth will have the psychological and social resources with which to cope with these adverse events and will never develop depressive symptoms or maladaptive behavior. A supportive family environment, for example, is a particularly strong resource from which a transgender youth can draw to sustain themselves through adversity [30]. For some transgender youth, stressors will overwhelm, at least temporarily, their capacity for resilience. Whether due to gender-affirming interventions or freedom to seek out less stigmatizing environments, transgender young adults tend to find themselves less victimized, more supported, and less depressed [26].

The cases below follow three transgender youths' exploration of their unique gender identities, experiences of internal and external stress related to their minority identity, and journey to understand their emerging identity and role in their school, community, and family. Each, for their own reasons, has suffered depressive feelings which have led to self-injury and/or suicidal behavior. As the following case discussions will point out, mental health professionals may employ different interventions at different times, with the focus being to help both youth and families face their angst rather than act it out, and clarify their emerging identity.

Case Reports

Case 1: Margarita

Margarita is a 16-year-old natal female, who presents for evaluation with their mother at a Midwestern university medical center-based Gender Evaluation Clinic. They are a warm, mature, polite, and thoughtful teenager, dressed in loose-fitting androgynous clothing with a very short haircut and no makeup. They describe their gender identity as "gender fluid/non-binary – I have not bothered to define it more than that," dating back to at least the seventh grade. They prefer to go by the name Marcos, due to its androgynous quality, and prefer the pronouns they or them, but would rather not be called she or her. Interestingly, they are comfortable with their mother referring to them as Margarita, adding: "That is what I am—her daughter. My birth name, Margarita, is kind of like an attachment between us. It would be weird for her to use any other name." Regarding therapy, Marcos confides that, "my personal goal is to become more comfortable with myself, and not have to change things about myself. Maybe even becoming comfortable with my birth name and female pronouns."

Diagnosis and Assessment: Case 1

During their first evaluation, Marcos declares that they are not interested in surgical interventions or hormonal interventions, stating "I am not uncomfortable with my body." They did not have difficulty, for example, when they went through puberty, although at times they will bind their breasts when they feel like looking more male. They also worry that because of their non-binary/gender-fluid identity, if they were to transition or do anything irreversible, they might later regret it. In general, Marcos feels very excited about their future and looks forward to going to college; they have a "pile" of recruitment information from the nation's best colleges. They hope to study law and are interested in social justice.

Marcos is currently a junior at an excellent Midwestern public high school, where they are thriving, taking many advanced placement and honors classes, with a high GPA and high PSAT scores. They are popular and celebrated in school, with supportive peers and teachers interested in learning about their non-binary identity. The school newspaper interviewed them regarding how to best use pronouns and labels for gender-variant youth. They have found much support at their school's GLOW group, "Gay, Lesbian, or Whatever!" Their impoverished family is from Colombia; their father was deported due to domestic violence, including beating their mother in their presence and threatening to rape his daughters. Their mother works as a cook in a Mexican diner and speaks only Spanish.

Marcos has had a nonconforming gender role and gender expression for their entire life. As a child, they always disliked dresses but did play with both girl and boy toys. Their mother states that in retrospect she suspected that her child was not comfortable with her gender, as she always rejected more feminine things and seemed to prefer masculine and boy-like things. Marcos states that fortunately their mother did not force them to wear dresses. Mother hopes to better understand what has caused this desire in her daughter to not be a girl and how she should respond as a mother.

In approximately the seventh grade, Marcos noticed that they yearned for things that were more typically boy or male and wished that girls would be allowed to enjoy such things. These feelings intensified, and in their sophomore year, they started "examining gender more." At that time they decided that they "sometimes feel more like a boy, but I am not a boy, and sometimes I feel more like a girl, but I am also not entirely a girl." This led to the realization that the gender label that seemed to make the most sense for them was non-binary or "gender fluid."

Marcos describes themselves as "pansexual," defining this as not being attracted to any specific gender, but rather a person. When they first "came out" to their mother during a therapy session as pansexual approximately a year ago, their mother started to cry, wondering if it was a genetic predisposition, since they have a gay uncle. Marcos replied, "Why are you crying about who I am?" Prior to that session, Marcos had become increasingly depressed and anxious with periods of suicidal ideation. The onset of their depression and anxious preoccupation was in their sophomore year when they started to examine sexuality and gender, coming to the conclusion that they were pansexual. They started to define as non-binary after making friends with a non-binary peer and learning of the existence of this category. However, they became increasingly saddened about losing their experience of growing up as a strong girl, wondering "Can I not be a feminist anymore, and is my childhood experience worthless, if I'm a guy or non-binary?" This led to an existential crisis with worsening mood and anxiety symptoms, and intensifying suicidal ideation, ultimately being placed on an SSRI trial along with starting supportive therapy with a bilingual therapist. Marcos states that their angst comes from "within." Although no longer depressed, they continue to wonder: "Who am I, and who am I going to be in life. There have been strong independent women who have helped me and raised me, like my mother, and if I am not a woman or girl, then who am I?" They continue to worry that by transitioning to a male or non-binary gender, they might be betraying the strong women who have helped them such as their mother, and they struggle with any identification that could put them closer to the neglectful and abusive men in their lives, such as their father. "The guys in my life have been crappy, so I don't want to be like them at all."

Management: Case 1

Over time their mood has brightened and the self-destructive urges subsided. Their non-binary gender identity has solidified, and they felt less ashamed of themselves and more able to share this aspect of their identity with their mother. When Marcos decided to share with mother their gender-fluid identity, "I eased mom into it. I have been starting to wear more guy stuff so that she would not be so surprised." However, they also "Sometimes still wonder where did I come from, and I start to feel useless. I will never hurt myself because I never want to hurt my mother, but then mom worries if she is not around, I won't have anything to live for." Mom became quite tearful when hearing this, admitting that it terrifies her to be the sole reason that her daughter will not act on their suicidal urges. Both mother and daughter admit that they survived their abusive father/husband by reaching out to each other, leaving them intertwined and scarred by their shared past trauma, and very much in need of mother-daughter family therapy.

A parent-child psychotherapy session was conducted at a follow-up session with the help of an interpreter. Marcos' mother was able to warmly and at times tearfully share with her daughter her many worries, but repeated that she loves her daughter more than anything on earth, that she loves her unconditionally and will always love her. She voiced her pride for how intelligent her child is and her belief that her child will do great things. Her daughter shared how meaningful it was to hear this unconditional support. Marcos' mother voiced that she feels so thankful that they are living in the United States, as this is a far more accepting and tolerant society versus the country they left behind. She has worked hard to overcome her tradition-bound cultural biases, in order to see her child as who *they* are.

Case 2: Sally

Diagnosis and Assessment: Case 2

Sally is a 14-year-old natal female, hospitalized for increasing depression and an overdose, triggered by his male gym teacher taunting him for not being able to do "push-ups like a guy." Sally states that his depression has worsened due to a deep lifelong conviction that he is a boy. He states that he has always felt like a boy and vividly recalls feeling like a boy in the first grade. He hated girl toys such as Barbie dolls, hated the color pink, and preferred playing with "other boys." Sally prefers the pronouns he/him/his, and has a private preferred male name that he will not share with others, for fear of rejection. His preferred and private male name was inspired by a favorite character from video games.

His parents, however, recall their child as gender nonconforming and vividly recall stretches of time when she was happy to be a girl, dressing as a girl and playing with girl toys. (Her parents continue to use female pronouns.) Parents believe that this gender dysphoria waned in the subsequent years; however, it intensified 1 year ago at the age of 13, when Sally started to assert that he was a boy and voice his desire for pubertal blockade to his parents and outpatient psychiatrist.

Sally's history is complicated with a period of severe depression leading to an overdose on aspirin and fluoxetine (prescribed for the depression) and a month-long stay on an inpatient unit. At that time Sally presented as an androgynous girl, with loose clothing, tousled shoulder-length hair, and no makeup.

Sally maintains an androgynous look, phenotypically presenting as female, and all who meet him assume he is a girl. He hates his breast development but does not bind and instead wears baggy clothes. He dreads further pubertal changes and wishes his parents would allow pubertal blockade. When asked why he does not do more to socially transition to a phenotypic male, he states that he cannot tolerate the thought of the teasing and scapegoating that he anticipates in his small town and school. He plans on shifting to a male gender role/expression when he goes to college, which gives him much hope. Several years after this hospitalization, Sally declared: "Eventually, I'm going to transition, which I probably am going to do. But I would want to be on the down low about it."

Management: Case 2

Inpatient DBT led to Sally gaining new skills to cope with her anger and depression rather than acting them out in self-injurious fashion, and his self-esteem improved. Interestingly, Sally was seen as a girl by all of his peers. He never corrected them.

He is extremely intelligent (scoring in the 99% on the standardized state exams) and tends to intellectualize most issues. He commented on his love of science, math, and facts and his love of Minecraft, adding: "It's cool that you can take a fence post and a door, and have them become a grandfather clock." When the psychiatrist commented on this striking transformation, similar to other desired transformations in life, Sally brightened and responded "Yes, a metaphor!"

A family meeting was held on the inpatient unit, in which his father tearfully asserted that he and his wife will certainly support their child regardless, and that if indeed *she* (italics used for parents' preferred pronouns) is a transgender child, they will do their best to *support her*. He and his wife feel that their daughter is not clear on *her* gender and that this might be yet another intense life phase, as *she* has had many dramatic moments in *her* life. They worry that this is simply another chapter in *her* struggle to consolidate *her* identity. They worry about doing anything that might lead to further difficulties down the road of life if *she* is not a truly a trans person. *Her* mother felt that a non-binary gender identity or even a gender-fluid one seems to better fit the child they know—Sally strongly rejects this option. Over time, however, *her* mother has become convinced that her child truly has a male gender identity and become supportive of her transitioning, a sentiment not shared by *her* father.

One year following discharge, Sally remains firm in his resolve to transition to a man when he enters college but is more accepting of his parents wanting to wait for hormonal interventions. His mother is willing to meet with the endocrinologist to learn more about reversible pubertal blockade; however, his father is very reluctant to support this. Sally's father remains skeptical regarding whether his child is a truly trans child and continues to feel that at most a gender-fluid label makes more sense, sharing that at times Sally will wear more feminine shirts and grow their hair out. He is also perplexed by *her* romantic interest in boys, which he feels does not support a transgender status. He has often said that "Sally's story is yet to be told." Father wonders about the impact of increased media exposure to transgendered people in shaping his child's gender identity. He deeply fears that medical interventions—such as pubertal blockade—might limit Sally's ability to appreciate the feminine and gender-conforming aspects of *herself*.

When asked about gender during a follow-up outpatient evaluation, Sally shared "I think of myself as male at least since 2014. When I was a little girl, though, I hated Barbie Dolls and pink, and I hated all that girl stuff. I went from a gender non-conforming girl to thinking of myself as male." He still does not correct others who refer to him as a girl, but he hates it that he does not pass as male. He vented that in choir he is required to wear long black skirts and tight black blouses with the girls, whereas the other boys "get to wear cool black tuxedos. Why can't it be like marching band where we all get to wear the same uniforms?" He wonders why we need to "distinguish the feminine."

He adds that his parents have been highly supportive and have not made transphobic or homophobic comments. "Even though my dad does not understand it, he just wants me to be happy. I am very lucky." Sally shared his conviction that her parents have confused sexual orientation with gender identity: "They thought I was doing this to get girls, and I do not even like girls! My dad thought I was a lesbian. I am attracted to guys and think of myself as a gay guy."

Sally went on: "What is gender? A social construct. For my purposes, I identify as male, I just do not get why that is a big deal. I would like to physically transition after 18, because my parents likely will not let me do it before then." He hopes for a mastectomy and gender reassignment surgery, as he despises his female anatomy and menses. Sally has found much acceptance from his peer group and teachers at school, especially an openly gay music teacher. Sally has shared with several close friends his "transguy" identity, and all have been supportive. Sally states the so-called bathroom bill in North Carolina mandating that individuals use bathrooms consistent with their assigned/natal gender, and not with their gender identity, is "ridiculous." Sally just does not understand why people need to make such a big deal of it, as most will never realize a person is trans; however, a number of their school peers have made comments against allowing transgender individuals to use bathrooms consistent with their gender identity. Sally wants to transition to being a typical guy and fears the stigma if one does not readily pass as the affirmed gender.

Sally does agree that stigma and shame have played a powerful role in his own life and impacted adjustment to his transgender identity. When asked to define what stigma meant to them, Sally states: "Social forces exerted onto you that make your situation more difficult." However, Sally is quite aware that the cost of "her" "passing" as cisgender and not transgender, to avoid awkward situations or stigma, comes at a price, as it is quite difficult to maintain such a front in the service of reducing stigma.

Sally adds that it is very difficult for him to see photos of himself. "I like my appearance, but I don't like that it does not reflect who I am, or what I see myself as." He yearns to be a traditional phenotypic male. He does not just wish for male attributes—he feels that his inner being is male and that his body does not reflect this. When asked about his Internet gaming presence, Sally states, "I say that I'm male, and it's really nice. Most of my friends are trans."

Sally links the onset of his depression to an intensification of his emerging awareness of being a boy and his related frustration over the stigma that he feared he would endure as a transman. Regarding the impact of his gender issues on the depression, Sally states, "the issues I was having with gender made the depression worse, but it was not just because of that, because depression also runs in my family, and it's biological. I am now on medication, and I'm not depressed, and I still feel exactly the same about my gender, so in that way it is not related." He feels hopeful that things will get better with time and pleased that his parents have brought him to a Gender Program.

Sally asserts that he does not want to shave the hair on his legs or elsewhere and that "if others were bothered by it, that was their problem." Her mother stated she was fine with this, but wanted her to know that this would put her at risk for teasing by others, to which Sally responded: "I like my body." Mother was pleased with this, as in the past she has stated that she does not like her body. More recently, Sally has been less focused on being trans, although he has clearly maintained a male gender identity/gender expression, sporting a new short haircut and unshaved legs.

After the psychiatrist commented on how being trans seemed a bit less central, Sally jokingly retorted: "The fact that I enjoy The Matrix Trilogy is more important than the fact that I am transgendered. And I only saw it once!"

In summary, Sally is a 14-year-old natal female, with a history of masculine and feminine play interests and a nonconforming female gender identity, who began to strongly identify as male at the age of 12. This male gender identity has persisted, and he yearns for hormonal and surgical interventions to become "a guy." His gender dysphoria has worsened during puberty. He rejects a "trans" or non-binary identity, and does not want to be a public figure or a "trans success story," which is why he is so very covert about his identity now and tolerates being seen as a girl. In contrast, he hopes to transition to "just being a gay guy" once he moves away to college. He is extremely intelligent, and prone to periods of anxiety and depression, including becoming severely depressed at the age of 14, leading to a suicide attempt by overdose and hospitalization. His mood has improved with treatment (antidepressant and psychotherapy), and his desire to transition to being a male has continued to intensify, though with continued expression of some feminine traits as well. His father, in particular, worries that given his identity shifts over time, gender transitioning interventions could shift the natural course of his gender identity. Ultimately, they are very supportive and want their child to be happy.

It is interesting that Sally tolerates being seen as a girl, due to his desire to avoid an "awkward situation." His parents wonder if it is more than that, believing that Sally still sometimes seems to enjoy being a girl at times, sometimes wearing more feminine sweaters, for example. They wonder if Sally might be a child with a non-binary or gender-fluid identity, with father convinced that she has not consolidated her identity in general, let alone her gender identity, and that her current trans status is a result of the forces of popular culture. Nevertheless, based on the intensity of his ongoing gender dysphoria, which has worsened during puberty, pubertal blockade was suggested to lessen some of the distress driven by development of secondary sex characteristics. Mother has been supportive of this, but father has not.

Sally was diagnosed with gender dysphoria and major depressive disorder, severe, in early remission. His depression was assessed to stem from both a positive family history and the impact of environmental stress such as stigma, and not simply an outgrowth of his gender dysphoria. He responded nicely to psychopharmacological intervention, coupled with ongoing therapy.

Case 3: Burt

Diagnosis and Assessment: Case 3

Burt is an 18-year-old natal female who prefers male pronouns such as he, him, or his and has a male gender identity. He was accompanied for the evaluation by his father, a police officer, and his mother, a teacher. His goal for the evaluation is to obtain support for his gender transitioning. He was neatly and casually dressed, wearing a camo-style male shirt, jeans, boy's boots, and a baseball style hat with a Pheasants Forever emblem. He presents as a phenotypic male, wearing a chest binder under his shirt, with the receptionist referring to him as a boy when she informed me that he was in the waiting room. He hopes to start hormonal treatment, specifically testosterone. He states that he has a firmly male gender identity but that he currently feels he is at a "standstill." "I am trying the hardest that I can to look like a male with no hormones, but I am really interested in moving forward with hormonal treatments." He is fine being referred to as a "guy, trans, or F to M."

Burt also shares that he yearns for "top surgery," so he will no longer have to bind his breasts daily. He tries not to look at his body, as it distresses him to see his female body. He states that he is relieved that he often does not have a period due to birth control. He is not interested in "bottom surgery" based on his research on the poor outcomes.

When asked about the evolution of his current gender identity, he states that he has had a firmly male gender identity for a long time but that he has not specifically thought of himself as a guy lifelong. Burt states that he has always hated feminine toys, clothing, or other things associated with being a girl. He has always been a tomboy and realizes that this must have been hard on his mother, who reportedly very much wanted "a little girl to do her hair, but I just did not like that at all."

He qualifies this by stating "when I was younger, I knew nothing about the LGBT community. I did not know about lesbian or gay people or trans people." Burt grew up in a small Midwestern town and states that he simply had no exposure to these various categories. He began to wonder about his sexuality when he was a freshman in high school while on the girls' volleyball team where he became emotionally and sexually drawn to a girl on the team. He began to wonder "what it was to like someone of my own sex. I did not even know about the existence of lesbians or gays and had never heard of that."

He began to learn more about different gender options and other sexual minorities by spending time looking at various YouTube channels. Two years ago, through YouTube, he first learned about transgender identity. He states "I initially wondered about maybe being simply gender fluid or non-binary, because I really did not want to be trans because all of the problems that go with being trans, but I just finally could not deny it any more. About a year ago, I decided that I am definitely a guy and trans."

At that time, Burt came out to his parents in the form of a letter. He researched how to come out to your parents online through various YouTubers and thought deeply about what would be the best way to go about doing this. He decided to write a letter, adding that he rewrote it at least seven times. His parents later shared the letter, and it is included verbatim below:

> Dear mom and dad, I could not get up the courage to say this in person. I did not want to see sad or confused looks on your faces, or have you tell me this is a phase and I do not know what I want or who I am. For the past 17 years, I have been your little girl. I have never felt comfortable, and I never knew why. Well … now I do. <u>I AM TRANS</u>. I am a boy in a girls' [sic] body. I know this is probably hard for you both. Mom, I know you wanted a daughter who would dress nice and pretty and do their hair and makeup and I tried being that for you,

> but it did not make me happy. Dad, I know this means I won't [sic] be "daddy's little girl" anymore, but can't I be daddy's little boy? I understand if you guys are sad or upset or confused. This is not a decision I made in a day. I have been thinking about this for LONG time. I am sorry I could not be the daughter you dreamed of. I hope from now on I can be the best son ever.

He placed the letter for his parents to see, and a few days passed. When his parents mentioned the letter, they were supportive, but admitted that it was very hard to comprehend what he was seeking from them. They worried about changing his name and gender too quickly, lest this all be a passing phase. Nevertheless, his father immediately started to research transgender youth and transition options including hormonal interventions and name change issues. They asked him to give them some time to agree upon a new name, reminding him how long it took to choose his natal female name. His parents also later admitted that they were surprised and hurt that he did not directly discuss this with them sooner. Burt shares that his parents and most family members remain incredibly supportive, referring to him as "Burt" or "their son." When others use his prior name or use a female pronoun, his dad will quickly correct them and say something such as "do you mean, Burt?" He is quite aware, however, that this has been extremely difficult for his parents.

Burt considered the possibility that he is not transgender but instead a lesbian and was even encouraged to explore a lesbian identity by his loving parents. He came to the deep conviction that this is not at all who he is, because he is simply a "guy." His identity is not just about his sexuality, and although he is primarily and predominantly attracted to girls, he does not consider himself a lesbian.

When asked about peers, Burt states "my friends understand completely, and have treated me very well." His cisgender male friends simply act like he is one of them now, and everyone at school now sees him as "Burt" and as "a guy," with no teasing whatsoever. The school nurse has been particularly understanding and helpful. He states "we can use the nurses' offices' bathrooms, or any bathroom that we choose in school, but for F to M's like me, the boys' bathroom had all the stalls ripped out so it is not so easy to use."

Burt has always been very athletic and involved in a number of sports teams, all of which were girls' teams when he was seemingly identified as a girl. However, he pulled out after socially transitioning to male and did not want to attempt to be on the boys' baseball team as it is an entirely different sport than girl's softball.

Burt has a brother who is about 5 years older and has largely been quite supportive. The two of them work out together and did have an awkward experience at a local gym. Burt was using the male bathroom and locker room when a staff member oddly approached him and asked him about "a problem" on his application. The staff member then interrogated him about his gender and name, stating that his name was a female and the gender was listed as female on the application, and therefore he simply could not use the male facilities. His mother later went to the fitness center and confronted the staff, who were very apologetic. His dad e-mailed the company's headquarters, who issued a letter of apology and support. Nevertheless, Burt was so upset that he withdrew his application.

Burt is looking forward to going to college following high school graduation. His father is investigating all options, including gender-neutral housing options. The school has been very supportive, although it is unclear how they will be assigning his roommate. Burt is hoping for a male roommate.

Burt's parents were interviewed following the interview with their son and presented as very loving and supportive parents. Burt's parents do not ever recall Burt saying that they wished they were a boy as a young child. (Burt remembers as a young child telling his older brother that he wanted to be a boy but later retracted this when his brother shared this with his parents.) They state that, in retrospect, Burt has always been very masculine and boy-like—for example, always wearing his older brother's clothes, including his underwear. He was very active and very involved in athletic teams and activities and never presented as a stereotypical feminine girl. About 2 years ago, around age 16, Burt casually mentioned that (at that point) she was "dating" somebody. When her parents asked who she was dating, she mentioned the name of a girl. Parents recall being very supportive of her romantic involvement at the time and thought of her as a lesbian. With the intervening events, they now realize that they have always had a son, but they just did not know it. His parents are supportive of his transitioning to a boy, including hormonal and surgical options. They are interested in consulting with pediatric endocrinology. Burt's parents agree the school has been very supportive, with the principal reaching out to them when he asked to be called Burt, to make sure the parents were comfortable with this.

Burt's journey of developing his identity was complicated by depression when he was a high school freshman, likely linked to coming to terms with his "sexuality/gender identity." During that time, he had a period of time when he was increasingly unhappy, with anhedonia, decreased energy, decreased concentration, decreased appetite, periods of mild agitation, and increased sleep. He never had thoughts of suicide or suicide attempts, but he engaged in non-suicidal self-injurious behavior (cutting) for a brief period of time, after learning about this option from a peer. Parents add that when they learned of the cutting they intervened immediately, telling Burt that it was not an acceptable option to hurt themselves. They sought consultation from his pediatrician who referred them to see a psychiatrist. The psychiatrist prescribed a course of an antidepressant, which the family stopped after a month. Burt's mood certainly brightened thereafter and he has not had any significant depression since that time. He also no longer cuts or injures himself in any way, and his mood remains bright.

To sum up, Burt is an 18-year-old natal female with a firmly male gender identity who presents in consultation hoping to be offered evaluation through pediatric endocrinology for hormonal interventions. He appears to be a very well-adjusted, articulate, and mature individual who has thought deeply about his gender identity and sexuality. Burt has a firmly held conviction that he is indeed a boy, rather than a girl or non-binary individual who simply wishes for aspects more typically acceptable for males in our society. Burt tried hard to take on a lesbian identity, or even a gender-fluid identity, understanding that either would possibly be an "easier" path to follow, but realized that he was not being true to "himself." He is incredibly fortunate to have understanding and nourishing parents who have done all they can to support their child in their search of a clearer sense of their identity.

Burt is indeed an adolescent with a persisting male gender identity and persisting gender dysphoria who has already socially transitioned to being a male over the past year. Burt presents as a phenotypic boy and would not be perceived as a girl by most individuals. Indeed, the receptionist at the front desk referred to him as a young man. His mannerisms are quite masculine, as are his hair style and clothing, and he binds his breasts daily. His dysphoria did increase during puberty, as is often seen in adolescents with persisting gender dysphoria. He is bothered by his female attributes and yearns for a body that reflects his underlying gender identity. When he socially transition to a boy, his depression and cutting both remitted, as has been described in the literature.

It is unlikely that these issues stem from another condition. He has no history of significant trauma or other comorbidities, apart from a period of depression likely related to the struggle of consolidating a stigmatized identity. His depression was mild and in no way has impacted his identity. He openly articulates that he tried hard to avoid taking on an identity which he realizes is complicated and rejected by many. Fortunately, he has had remarkable acceptance by his peers and staff at school, where he has seamlessly transitioned to being registered as a boy, and by his family, including his grandparents, brother, and extended family. All this bodes well for an excellent adjustment as he fully transitions to becoming a man.

His parents are appropriately worried about the turbulence he will likely encounter in the future and particularly worry about when he will be at college away from their immediate protection. They have appropriately intervened with the college, making certain the school is supportive of gender-nonconforming and transgender youth. Both parents now celebrate their son and have moved past mourning the loss of a daughter.

Management: Case 3

Burt is a good candidate for hormonal interventions, specifically testosterone, and was referred to our pediatric endocrinologist. Burt was thrilled, as he has been hoping for this for a very long time. Burt and his parents agreed to follow up the Gender Program for ongoing consultation. Psychotherapy was recommended for Burt as a forum where he can explore other aspects related to his identity and work through some of the difficult situations he will likely encounter due to societal intolerance toward trans individuals. Burt has also been very thoughtful about the future and states that he would like to be a dad someday. He is interested in preserving eggs before starting testosterone, to maintain the option of having children in this way versus adoption. This future-oriented stance also bodes well for his psychological adjustment and his capacity to effectively consolidate his identity.

Table 11.2 presents characteristics of the three cases discussed.

Table 11.2 Case characteristics

	Marcos	Sally	Burt
Natal gender	Female	Female	Female
Gender identity	Non-binary	Male	Male
Preferred pronouns	"They-them-theirs"	"He-him-his"	"He-him-his"
Mood at evaluation	Euthymic	Intensely dysphoric	Euthymic
Suicide risk at evaluation	Low to moderate	High	Low
Referral for gender-affirming medical interventions	None	Delayed	Immediate

Clinical Pearls/Pitfalls

Why Is Gender Such a Big Deal?

This chapter explores the co-occurrence of depression, self-injury, and suicide among transgender youth. Clinical samples suggest that transgender youth are at more risk than their cisgender peers of experiencing depression, self-injurious behavior, and suicide. While the majority will *not* experience these challenges, a significant minority will. The cases presented in this chapter illustrate how depression and even self-injury and suicidal thinking occur within an individual context that must be explored. Clues arise from the case discussions as to the context predisposing transgender youth to developing depression and self-directed violence. A discussion of this context captures the answer to the second objective for this chapter: understanding the current theoretical framework for depression arising in transgender youth.

While the concept of assigned "gender" and its relationship to one's anatomical sex is easy to describe, the meaning attributed to gender—and to behaviors not conforming to one's assigned gender—is much more fluid between individuals and cultures. Transgender youth, willingly or not, have been thrust into a polarizing political battle recently in the United States, as cultures around the world struggle with the acceptance of gender minorities.

Infants as early as 12 months show sex-specific toy preferences along socially prescribed gender stereotypes, preschool children as early as age 3 are able to recognize their own and others' sex, and school-age children show a clear gender preference for playmates [31]. Patterns of gender expression are appreciable throughout childhood (reviewed by Steensma et al. [32]). Most children will conform to societal expectations regarding their natal gender, while others will display incongruence. Most of these gender-nonconforming children will settle into their natal gender by adolescence (but may take on a sexual minority identity later) [33, 34]. Even so, gender nonconformity throughout childhood can lead to stress as children and families develop within a society with strict gender roles, as captured in all three cases. Unfortunately, mounting evidence suggests that in the United States, gender nonconformity in childhood makes children more prone to bullying and abuse [27]. Such hostile environments can have immediate and long-lasting psychological effects. Marcos' case demonstrates how early adversity from within and outside the family can contribute to later depression, in keeping with both retrospective and longitudinal studies [27, 35, 36] while at the same time providing a shared experience of trauma that strengthened support from their mother. Despite legal efforts by the United Nations and other international agencies, gender-nonconforming children living in many parts of the world grow up with even more exposure to victimization than in the United States and can face victimization from multiple sources during the immigration process [37]. Victimization and prejudice is not limited to childhood and has been postulated to play a key role in the development of psychological maladjustment including depressive symptoms and self-directed violence among sexual and gender minorities [38].

For transgender youth, not all stress originates from external sources. Compared to natal girls, natal boys strive harder to conform to gender role expectations, increasing internal stress for those displaying gender incongruence [12, 39]. Around ages 10–13, most children will gain more traits congruent with their natal gender, widening the gap between gender-conforming and nonconforming behaviors [32]. Adolescence is a time for exploration and consolidation of multiple facets of identity. This seems to be no different for gender, as both cisgender and transgender teens have been found to explore and appreciate both masculine and feminine aspects of themselves related to peer interactions and social context. Such exploration likely leads to a rich diversity of cisgender males with some feminine traits and cisgender females with some masculine traits [40]. In this context, Sally's intermittent desire to wear his hair long, wear more feminine clothing, and keep a public female name does not necessarily imply that his core gender identity is anything other than "a guy." In his words, he even sometimes finds it irritating or semantic to "distinguish the feminine." Ultimately, as Sally and Burt both describe, their transgender identity runs much deeper than hair or clothing. Transgender youth like those described above do not just wish for some traits of another gender but have within them an essential belief of *being* another gender [41, 42]. Sally also captures the desire common among youth that they not be reduced to any one aspect of their identities. Being a transboy is just *part* of who he is, as captured many years ago in the seminal work of Goffman examining the tendency to reduce individuals to the stigmatized aspects of themselves [43].

Youth (and families) can experience this variability in gender expression as dissonant to society's expectations about gender identity. Keenly aware of the consequences of settling into such a stigmatized identity, teenagers can try to hide this aspect of themselves to avoid detection. Marcos, Sally, and Burt all experienced dysphoria around the time they recall exploring their identities as trans, even before they disclosed this identity to anyone. In these cases, dysphoria likely revolved around the process of acquiring a stigmatized identity, which in their cases included self-stigmatization and efforts to hide their identities from others. *Transphobia* denotes the fear and prejudice against individuals who do not conform to societal expectations of identity, mannerisms, speech, dress, and other aspects of gender expression [44]. *Internalized transphobia* describes a defense mechanism within the individual to resolve tension about societal rules and personal desires [45], in which a transgender individual holds these societal attitudes within him/herself, in many cases leading to profound self-shaming, anticipation and fear of shaming by others, and a motivation for self-directed violence. Burt faced an early struggle after realizing a core aspect of his identity was one that society stigmatized and described a period of depression and cutting prior to disclosing to his family and others his transgender identity. Burt recalled this as a time when "….I really did not want to be trans because all of the problems that go with being trans, but I just finally could not deny it anymore." Perez-Brumer et al. [46] found that internalized transphobia was correlated with lifetime suicide attempts among a sample of transgender adults in the United States, and Marshall et al. [47] found a similar correlation among transgender adults in Argentina. Some research has focused on how gender minorities have dealt with transphobia as the key to unlocking why some transgender youth experience more emotional distress than others. Hatzenbuehler, for example, has hypothesized that the ways in which minority youth cope with their stigmatized role could mediate psychological distress (reviewed in [48]). Others, such as Goffman, have focused on youth dismissing and denying their stigmatized identity [43, 49]. To avoid shame and stigma, some youth use "impression management" skills—as is borne out in the cases above. Sally has tried to "pass" with his natal female gender to avoid a stigmatizing transgender identity, for example, by letting others refer to him by the female name Sally. While this strategy seems adaptive, it comes at a cost for most youth, as the constant self-monitoring employed to avoid acting *too* different usually leads to fear, isolation, poor self-esteem, and feelings of worthlessness [49]. The torment growing out of Sally's internal conflict about his social transition and his need to maintain a "down low" secrecy, Marcos' existential struggle at recognizing their non-binary identity, and Burt's depression while silently accepting his minority identity are examples of how the process of taking on a stigmatized identity can impact clinical depressive symptoms and self-directed violence.

While all transgender individuals within a society will experience the same large-scale shifts in culture toward acceptance or rejection, and while many will experience at least some of the internal psychological consequences of these shifts, only a minority will develop depressive symptoms and be at risk of self-injury and suicide. The third focal point of the chapter is that of the resilience in spite of social challenges that is afforded by families embracing their transgender child, allowing them to explore their emerging gender identity.

On a smaller scale than prevailing social attitudes and victimization of transgender youth, ongoing research demonstrates the importance of acceptance and rejection within the family. As demonstrated in the case examples, just as structure differs family to family, so too does the degree of acceptance and rejection of the gender-nonconforming child. Burt describes his family as having been extremely accepting of the sexual and gender aspects of his identity, Sally has struggled with his perceived minimization of his stated gender by his family, and Marcos (Margarita to her mother) has seen their mother as their core support, to the point that they wonder how they would go on living without her. The best mental health outcomes are indeed found when family support is matched by peer and other community supports [35]. These cases further bear out something consistent with the literature—that family acceptance and rejection often coexist, and although they are born out of parental attitudes, the child's interpretation of parental behavior is key [50]. That is, family acceptance and rejection are "in the eye of the beholder." Take, for example, Sally's description of his parents as "highly supportive" while at the same time having recognized some rejection as his parents, especially his father, still struggle to understand his gender identity. Rejection by family members has been shown to make transgender youth prone to negative health outcomes including depression and self-directed violence [29]. Parental rejection often does not arise from malice but instead may emerge from grieving the loss of the future they had fantasized for their child, fearing for the well-being of their child in a stigmatizing society, and feelings of shame and torment within themselves [51]. Clinical experience from a program specifically designed to help families accept their gender and sexual minority children indicates that most parents desire to improve their acceptance of their children [50].

Promoting Resiliency and Healing for Transgender Youth and Families: Concluding Thoughts

Sexual and gender minority youth, including gay, lesbian, bisexual, and transgender youth, and those with other creative and nonconforming ways of describing their gender and sexual selves are particularly vulnerable to several psychological and social stressors that subsequently predispose to depressive distress and self-directed violence. These stressors are particularly pronounced during the early and late adolescent years when the young person's development centers on making sense of one's gender, sexuality, and other aspects of one's identity [52]. Transgender youth face numerous struggles through the course of their childhood and adolescence, often because of their nonconforming gender identity, leading to much angst and putting some at heightened risk for clinical depressive disorders, anxiety disorders, and self-injurious behaviors. In most cases, transgender youth are resilient in the face of these stressors and will never need clinical help. For those who do present for treatment of depression, anxiety, and/or self-directed violence, the primary intervention is for the mental health professional to assess the degree of internal torment and investigate the sources of this discontent with respect to incongruence of anatomy and/or natal/assigned gender to experienced gender. Providers must consider contributing biological factors (e.g., major depression symptomatology, family history of major depression, or other mood disorders), stigmatization, victimization, family acceptance/rejection, shame, internalized transphobia, and impression management efforts in the evaluation of such youth.

The final objective of this chapter is a discussion of the rationale for treatment of depression in gender dysphoric youth, specifically with respect to referral for gender-affirming medical interventions such as pubertal blockade. In cases of a depressed transgender youth, the mental health clinician will most likely be asked to comment on the youth's mental status and capacity to consent for medical interventions such as puberty suppression or cross-sex hormones [53]. Referral for appropriate gender-affirming medical interventions should be considered, if appropriate, once the child's depression, for example, is in remission, or it is felt that the gender issues are driving the subsequent depression. Some depressed transgender youth like Marcos do not desire gender-affirming medical interventions, and the focus of treatment can remain on helping the adolescent consolidate a healthy identity while managing stigma, shame, depression, and self-directed violence. For those who do desire gender-affirming interventions, like Sally and Burt, some youths' depression and self-directed violence are so acute at the time of presentation that gender-affirming interventions are unlikely to succeed until the depression is treated. Using Sally's case as an example, his initial presentation—hospitalized following a potentially lethal suicide attempt—required immediate treatment with a combination of antidepressant medication and dialectical behavioral therapy to make it possible to transition to outpatient care and then to proceed with gender-affirming interventions. In contrast, Burt presented as having endured an episode of depression and engaged in non-suicidal self-injury in the past, but was euthymic at the time of presentation, making an immediate referral for medical interventions feasible. At times ascertaining how paramount pubertal physical changes incongruent to one's gender identity might be to the emergence of the depression is straightforward and at other times more complicated. For example, in Sally's case his firmly held gender identity did not shift once his depression remitted, and he clearly stated that his desire to be a boy was a driving force to his depression, suggesting that at least for some adolescents proceeding with gender-affirming interventions even before depression has remitted may be helpful. In other cases, youth may not initially know or be able to describe how incongruent pubertal changes have affected their mood.

The role of the mental health professional in the care of transgender youth is evolving with time [54], from the role of a gatekeeper to medical interventions to the role of supporting youth and their families through the transition process [55]. While no evidence-based guidelines exist regarding other interventions for depression among transgender youth, ongoing psychotherapy is vital, with psychotherapeutic interventions aimed at nonjudgmentally exploring identity, reducing internalized stigma and shame within the youth and the family, improving family and outside social support, promoting resilience when adversity arises, and instilling hope. These are reviewed in the American Academy of Child and Adolescent Psychiatry (AACAP) Practice Parameter for Assessment of Sexual and Gender Minorities [56] and in other texts (e.g., Leibowitz et al. [53]). Additionally, the American Academy of Child and Adolescent Psychiatry (AACAP) Practice Parameter for Treatment of Child and Adolescent Depression, while not specifically written with transgender youth in mind, should serve as a resource for guiding other psychotherapeutic and medical interventions for depressed youth [9]. As Leibowitz and de Vries [54] point out, a comprehensive assessment of gender dysphoric adolescents will also comprise of time spent with the entire family and time spent with the parent(s) alone. It is crucial that parents have a space to share their fears and struggles as well and work to gradually become more accepting of their transgender child in the service of protecting their child from negative outcomes including depression and self-directed violence. In the end, mental health professionals can ideally create a therapeutic space allowing youth and family members to embark on a journey together toward finding meaning in their gender identity, facilitating integration within their larger identities and lives.

References

1. de Vries ALC, Doreleijers TAH, Steensma TD, Cohen-Kettenis PT. Psychiatric comorbidity in gender dysphoric adolescents. J Child Psychol Psychiatry. 2011;52(11):1195–202.
2. Mustanski BS, Garofalo R, Emerson EM. Mental health disorders, psychological distress, and suicidality in a diverse sample of lesbian, gay, bisexual, and transgender youths. Am J Public Health. 2010;100(12):2426–32.
3. de Vries AL, McGuire JK, Steensma TD, Wagenaar EC, Doreleijers TA, Cohen-Kettenis PT. Young adult psychological outcome after puberty suppression and gender reassignment. Pediatrics. 2014;134(4):696–704.
4. Dhejne C, Van Vlerken R, Heylens G, Arcelus J. Mental health and gender dysphoria: a review of the literature. Int Rev Psychiatry. 2016;28(1):44–57.
5. Grossman AH, D'Augelli AR. Transgender youth and life-threatening behaviors. Suicide Life Threat Behav. 2007;37(5):527–37.
6. Arcelus J, Claes L, Witcomb GL, Marshall E, Bouman WP. Risk factors for non-suicidal self-injury among trans youth. J Sex Med. 2016;13(3):402–12.
7. Olson J, Schrager SM, Belzer M, Simons LK, Clark LF. Baseline physiologic and psychosocial characteristics of transgender youth seeking care for gender dysphoria. J Adolesc Health. 2015;57(4):374–80.
8. Control NCfIPa. 10 Leading Causes of Death, United States: 2014, All Races, Both Sexes: United States Centers for Disease Control and Prevention; 2014 [updated December 8, 2015; cited Centers for Disease Control and Prevention]. http://www.cdc.gov/injury/images/lc-charts/leading_causes_of_death_age_group_2014_1050w760h.gif.
9. Birmaher B, Brent D, Bernet W, Bukstein O, Walter H, Benson RS, et al. Practice parameter for the assessment and treatment of children and adolescents with depressive disorders. J Am Acad Child Adolesc Psychiatry. 2007;46(11):1503–26.
10. Spack NP, Edwards-Leeper L, Feldman HA, Leibowitz S, Mandel F, Diamond DA, et al. Children and adolescents with gender identity disorder referred to a pediatric medical center. Pediatrics. 2012;129(3):418–25.
11. Zucker KJ. Gender identity disorder in children and adolescents. Ann Rev Clin Psychol. 2005;1:467–92.
12. Yunger JL, Carver PR, Perry DG. Does gender identity influence children's psychological well-being? Dev Psychol. 2004;40(4):572–82.
13. Wallien MSC, Swaab H, Cohen-Kettenis PT. Psychiatric comorbidity among children with gender identity disorder. J Am Acad Child Adolesc Psychiatry. 2007;46(10):1307–14.
14. Singh D, Bradley SJ, Zucker KJ. Commentary on "an affirmative intervention for families with gender variant children: parental ratings of child mental health and gender" by hill, Menvielle, Sica, and Johnson (2010). J Sex Marital Therapy. 2011;37(2):151–7.

15. De Ceglie D, Freedman D, McPherson S, Richardson P. Children and adolescents referred to a specialist gender identity development service: clinical features and demographic characteristics: symposion; 2002. http://www.iiav.nl/ezines/web/ijt/97-03/numbers/symposion/ijtvo06no01_01.htm.
16. Feinleib MR, editor. Report of the secretary's task force on youth suicide. Rockville, MD: Alcohol Drug Abuse, and Mental Health Administration; 1989. p. 115.
17. Marshall E, Claes L, Bouman WP, Witcomb GL, Arcelus J. Non-suicidal self-injury and suicidality in trans people: a systematic review of the literature. Int Rev Psychiatry. 2016;28(1):58–69.
18. Holt V, Skagerberg E, Dunsford M. Young people with features of gender dysphoria: demographics and associated difficulties. Clin Child Psychol Psychiatry. 2016;21(1):108–18.
19. Skagerberg E, Parkinson R, Carmichael P. Self-harming thoughts and behaviors in a group of children and adolescents with gender dysphoria. Int J Transgender. 2013;14(2):86–92.
20. Plener PL, Libal G, Keller F, Fegert JM, Muehlenkamp JJ. An international comparison of adolescent non-suicidal self-injury (NSSI) and suicide attempts: Germany and the USA. Psychol Med. 2009;39(9):1549–58.
21. Aitken M, VanderLaan DP, Wasserman L, Stojanovski S, Zucker KJ. Self-harm and suicidality in children referred for gender dysphoria. J Am Acad Child Adolesc Psychiatry. 2016;55(6):513–20.
22. Reisner SL, Vetters R, Leclerc M, Zaslow S, Wolfrum S, Shumer D, et al. Mental health of transgender youth in care at an adolescent urban community health center: a matched retrospective cohort study. J Adolesc Health. 2015;56(3):274–9.
23. Kosciw JG, Greytak EA, Palmer NA, Boesen MJ. The 2013 National School Climate Survey: the experiences of lesbian, gay, bisexual, and transgender youth in our nation's schools. New York City, NY: GLSEN; 2014.
24. Claes L, Bouman WP, Witcomb G, Thurston M, Fernandez-Aranda F, Arcelus J. Non-suicidal self-injury in trans people: associations with psychological symptoms, victimization, interpersonal functioning, and perceived social support. J Sex Med. 2015;12(1):168–79.
25. Clements-Nolle K, Marx R, Katz M. Attempted suicide among transgender persons: the influence of gender-based discrimination and victimization. J Homosex. 2006;51(3):53–69.
26. Birkett M, Newcomb ME, Mustanski B. Does it get better? A longitudinal analysis of psychological distress and victimization in lesbian, gay, bisexual, transgender, and questioning youth. J Adolesc Health. 2015;56(3):280–5.
27. Roberts AL, Rosario M, Slopen N, Calzo JP, Austin SB. Childhood gender nonconformity, bullying victimization, and depressive symptoms across adolescence and early adulthood: an 11-year longitudinal study. J Am Acad Child Adolesc Psychiatry. 2013;52(2):143–52.
28. de Vries AL, Steensma TD, Cohen-Kettenis PT, VanderLaan DP, Zucker KJ. Poor peer relations predict parent- and self-reported behavioral and emotional problems of adolescents with gender dysphoria: a cross-national, cross-clinic comparative analysis. Eur Child Adolesc Psychiatry. 2016;25(6):579–88.
29. Ryan C, Huebner D, Diaz RM, Sanchez J. Family rejection as a predictor of negative health outcomes in White and Latino lesbian, gay, and bisexual young adults. Pediatrics. 2009;123(1):346–52.
30. Ryan C, Russell ST, Huebner D, Diaz R, Sanchez J. Family acceptance in adolescence and the health of LGBT young adults. J Child Adolesc Psychiatr Nurs. 2010;23(4):205–13.
31. Hines M. Prenatal endocrine influences on sexual orientation and on sexually differentiated childhood behavior. Front Neuroendocrinol. 2011;32(2):170–82.
32. Steensma TD, Kreukels BPC, de Vries ALC, Cohen-Kettenis PT. Gender identity development in adolescence. Horm Behav. 2013;64(2):288–97.
33. Wallien MSC, Cohen-Kettenis PT. Psychosexual outcome of gender-dysphoric children. J Am Acad Child Adolesc Psychiatry. 2008;47(12):1413–23.
34. Steensma TD, McGuire JK, Kreukels BP, Beekman AJ, Cohen-Kettenis PT. Factors associated with desistence and persistence of childhood gender dysphoria: a quantitative follow-up study. J Am Acad Child Adolesc Psychiatry. 2013;52(6):582–90.

35. McConnell EA, Birkett MA, Mustanski B. Typologies of social support and associations with mental health outcomes among LGBT youth. LGBT Health. 2015;2(1):55–61.
36. Nuttbrock L, Hwahng S, Bockting W, Rosenblum A, Mason M, Macri M, et al. Psychiatric impact of gender-related abuse across the life course of male-to-female transgender persons. J Sex Res. 2010;47(1):12–23.
37. Alessi EJ, Kahn S, Chatterji S. 'The darkest times of my life': recollections of child abuse among forced migrants persecuted because of their sexual orientation and gender identity. Child Abuse Negl. 2016;51:93–105.
38. Meyer IH. Prejudice, social stress, and mental health in lesbian, gay, and bisexual populations: conceptual issues and research evidence. Psychol Bull. 2003;129(5):674–97.
39. Egan SK, Perry DG. Gender identity: a multidimensional analysis with implications for psychosocial adjustment. Dev Psychol. 2001;37(4):451–63.
40. McHale SM, Kim JY, Dotterer AM, Crouter AC, Booth A. The development of gendered interests and personality qualities from middle childhood through adolescence: a biosocial analysis. Child Dev. 2009;80(2):482–95.
41. Daniolos PT. Gender identity: on being versus wishing. J Am Acad Child Adolesc Psychiatry. 2013;52(6):569–71.
42. Daniolos PT, Telingator CJ. Engendering identity. J Am Acad Child Adolesc Psychiatry. 2013;52(12):1245–7.
43. Goffman E. Stigma; notes on the management of spoiled identity. Englewood Cliffs, NJ: Prentice-Hall; 1963. p. 147.
44. Warriner K, Nagoshi CT, Nagoshi JL. Correlates of homophobia, transphobia, and internalized homophobia in gay or lesbian and heterosexual samples. J Homosex. 2013;60(9):1297–314.
45. Margolies L, Becker M, Jackson-Brewer K. Internalized homophobia: identifying and treating the oppressor within. In: Collectives B, editor. Lesbian psychologies: explorations and challenges. Chicago, IL: University of Illinois Press; 1987. p. 229–42.
46. Perez-Brumer A, Hatzenbuehler ML, Oldenburg CE, Bockting W. Individual- and structural-level risk factors for suicide attempts among transgender adults. Behav Med. 2015;41(3):164–71.
47. Marshall BD, Socias ME, Kerr T, Zalazar V, Sued O, Aristegui I. Prevalence and correlates of lifetime suicide attempts among transgender persons in Argentina. J Homosex. 2016;63(7):955–67.
48. Hatzenbuehler ML. How does sexual minority stigma "get under the skin"? A psychological mediation framework. Psychol Bull. 2009;135(5):707–30.
49. Radkowsky M, Siegel LJ. The gay adolescent: stressors, adaptations, and psychosocial interventions. Clin Psychol Rev. 1997;17(2):191–216.
50. SAMHSA (Substance Abuse and Mental Health Services Administration). A practitioner's resource guide: helping families to support their LGBT children (Contract No.: HS Publication No. PEP14-LGBTKIDS). Rockville, MD: Substance Abuse and Mental Health Services Administration; 2014.
51. Dierckx M, Motmans J, Mortelmans D, T'sjoen G. Families in transition: a literature review. Int Rev Psychiatry. 2016;28(1):36–43.
52. Erikson EH. Childhood and society. New York, NY: Norton; 1963.
53. Leibowitz S, Chen D, Marco AH. Gender dysphoria and nonconformity. In: Dulcan MK, editor. Dulcan's textbook of child and adolescent psychiatry. 2nd ed. Arlington, VA: American Psychiatric Association; 2016. p. 585–602.
54. Leibowitz S, de Vries AL. Gender dysphoria in adolescence. Int Rev Psychiatry. 2016;28(1):21–35.
55. Bockting WO. Vulnerability and resilience among gender-nonconforming children and adolescents: mental health professionals have a key role to play. J Am Acad Child Adolesc Psychiatry. 2016;55(6):441–3.
56. Adelson SL. Practice parameter on gay, lesbian, or bisexual sexual orientation, gender nonconformity, and gender discordance in children and adolescents. J Am Acad Child Adolesc Psychiatry. 2012;51(9):957–74.

Chapter 12
Gender Dysphoria and Psychotic Spectrum Disorders

Aron Janssen and Brandon S. Ito

Introduction

This chapter highlights the experience of Amy, a 20-year-old transgender female with diagnoses of schizoaffective disorder, gender dysphoria, marijuana use disorder, and a history of cocaine abuse who was initially referred to an outpatient gender and sexuality mental health clinic at age 17 for an evaluation of gender and sexual identity issues. This case hopes to illustrate the developmental pathway of an adolescent with gender dysphoria and psychosis, to examine unique challenges in treating patients with both psychotic spectrum disorders and gender dysphoria, and to highlight the frequent traumas transgender individuals' face as a part of their gender identity.

Brief Literature Review

Gender affirmative care is effective in diminishing gender dysphoria (GD) for 80% of individuals, and 78% of individuals with GD that receive gender affirmative care had significant improvement in co-occurring psychiatric symptoms, including those of depression, anxiety, substance abuse, and suicidality [1]. And yet, the very

A. Janssen, MD (✉)
Department of Child and Adolescent Psychiatry, NYU Langone Health, NYU Child Study Center, New York, NY, USA
e-mail: aron.janssen@nyumc.org

B. S. Ito, MD, MPH
Department of Psychiatry, UCLA Semel Institute for Neuroscience and Human Behavior, Los Angeles, CA, USA
e-mail: bito@mednet.ucla.edu

A. Janssen, S. Leibowitz (eds.), *Affirmative Mental Health Care for Transgender and Gender Diverse Youth*, https://doi.org/10.1007/978-3-319-78307-9_12

domains that can improve with appropriate treatment of GD are also those that represent barriers to accessing that care. According to the World Professional Association of Transgender Health Standards of Care, Version 7, co-occurring psychiatric symptoms must be "reasonably well-controlled" to access gender-affirming hormones and surgery. For episodic illnesses, the concept of assessing for reasonably well-controlled symptoms is easier to define; however, for chronic psychotic disorders, this becomes a much more complex task.

Historically, until the mid-twentieth century, transgender individuals were assumed to be severely mentally disturbed in order to want to access care. The prevailing opinion of that time was that GD could exist only within the context of severe personality disorders or psychosis [2, 3]. Over time, more research and clinical experience pointed toward complex psychiatric symptoms being result of untreated GD as opposed to the cause. Alternatively, others have suggested that the reason for the increased psychiatric symptoms seen in transgender individuals as compared to the general population is related to the minority stress and increased exposure to trauma, bullying, and rejection as a result of their identity. That is, daily exposure to stigma and bias (be it covert or overt) has significant long-term impact on the psychosocial outcomes of a minority community. For transgender youth who face increased risk of violence and rejection, we would expect to see increased rates of psychopathology in this population.

Despite these advances in understanding the relationship between psychiatric symptoms and GD, individuals with psychotic spectrum symptoms and GD are still often thought to have the GD stem from the psychosis as opposed to the psychosis and GD co-occurring independently of one another. Recent research demonstrates that rates of psychosis among individuals with GD are no higher than in the general population [4]. And yet, much of the contemporary literature about the overlap between psychosis and GD discusses the need for extreme caution in allowing patients to access care. In a study from 2001 [5], the author cautioned that schizophrenic patients commonly present behind a mask of GD for surgery. Other studies, while less overtly biased, have excluded patients from enrollment when psychotic symptoms were present, making it difficult to draw conclusions about the specific needs for this population. Specific concerns raised include the potential impact of hormone treatment on psychotic symptoms, the capacity to provide consent among those with psychosis, the possibility of impulsive decision-making and/or regret, and the availability of safe, stable housing for recovery. Unfortunately, data on most of these concerns is sparse and limited only to case studies in the literature.

Specifically related to masculinizing hormones, there is literature to suggest that unmonitored, high-dose anabolic steroid use can lead to psychotic symptoms [6]. However, most of the participants studied used metabolites of testosterone, rather than testosterone itself. Additionally, systematic review of the impact of hormones on the mental health of individuals with GD do not demonstrate any elevated levels of psychosis among participants [7]. That said, it is difficult to draw conclusions from this research—the data on high-dose testosterone derivatives is not analogous to the use of testosterone in GD, and many individuals with active psychosis have historically been unable to access hormonal care, so the number of individuals with chronic psychotic disorders in the systematic review is negligible. As for feminizing hormones, there is some evidence to suggest that estrogen is actually protective against psychosis in vulnerable individuals [8] and may explain why women have a later onset of initial symptoms of schizophrenia and why symptoms are exacerbated during low estrogen states. Again, we must be careful not to glean too much from this data, as systematic study of the impact of estrogen on individuals with both GD and psychosis has not been done.

However, more recent literature [9] has begun to compile case examples of the successful treatment of GD among the chronically psychotic population. These case studies have been able to demonstrate successful treatment with appropriate support.

In addition to the concern about the impact of gender-affirming care on the experience of psychiatric symptoms, there have also been concerns raised about the impact of psychiatric symptoms on the ability to follow through with the necessary steps for successful treatment, particularly for surgery. Historically, individuals with chronic psychotic symptoms have had their ability to consent to procedures underestimated by their medical providers. Many individuals with chronic psychotic symptoms are able to successfully navigate complex procedures and treatments with appropriate supports. However, there are occasional more complex structural barriers for individuals with psychosis that are independent of their mental illness that may impact ability to recovery from surgery. For example, many individuals with chronic psychotic symptoms lack stable housing and may have difficulty maintaining aftercare in a safe manner without support. In assessing all individuals for preparedness for surgery, but in particular those with chronic psychotic conditions, these potential structural barriers should be assessed and addressed as a part of the presurgical process.

Case Report

Amy began to identify as gay male at the age of 15 and struggled initially to come to terms with her sexuality. She found herself attracted emotionally and sexually exclusively to boys but found the label of gay didn't feel quite right. She had experienced some preferences for more stereotypically feminine interests and dress for a brief time in childhood but had never previously had thoughts about wishing she were or experiencing herself as a girl. Despite her discomfort with the label gay, and what it mean to her burgeoning gender identity, she nevertheless came out as gay to friends and family.

Her experience in coming out was met by conflict both at home and at school. At school in particular, she was constantly verbally assaulted by her classmates and was the victim of violence from peers. She became depressed at that time and began seeing both a psychologist and psychiatrist and treated with aripiprazole for a few months. Partly due to a rejection of her sexual orientation, she became estranged from her biological father whose parents had separated when she was a few months old. Later that year, she also experienced her first sexual assault by a person she had met through a popular phone dating application. She initially told nobody about the assault and began to withdraw socially and began using drugs and alcohol during the weekends and occasionally while at school.

At the age of 16 years, Amy was psychiatrically hospitalized for the first time for depression and concurrent cocaine abuse for 2 weeks and discharged on escitalopram. Amy defined her gender identity as "androgynous" during this time, occasionally dressing publicly in woman's clothing, wearing makeup and long-haired wigs. She used both male and female gendered names among different social groups. As a result of ongoing bullying, Amy transferred to a specialized school for LGBTQ youth during her junior year of high school; however, that year there was a notable decline in her academics to the point where she was barely able to advance to her senior year. She was unable to maintain regular outpatient psychiatric follow-up but engaged in two outpatient substance abuse rehab programs at the insistence of her family.

As she began to come to terms with her gender identity as that of a woman, she also sought sex hormone treatment for the first time; however, she was told that she would not be eligible for hormone treatment through the clinic until she turned 18 years of age. She was then referred to the child and adolescent psychiatry gender and sexuality specialty clinic for further evaluation of gender identity issues.

Following her initial evaluation in the gender and sexuality clinic, Amy was instructed to go to the emergency room for a psychiatric evaluation due to her family's concerns about her recent odd behavior and safety. In the emergency room, it was noted that increasingly over the past few months, Amy began to voice that someone was "tapping" her phone, using her social security number, and she frequently worried about the safety of her family. This was accompanied by a dramatic change in dress, use of excessive makeup, and vague statements about needing to leave the family to join a secret society to obtain fame and fortune. Other symptoms included ideas of reference through the radio and television. Amy also endorsed feelings of depression, sleeping excessively, having little pleasure in activities, poor energy, poor concentration, and decreased appetite with a 20-pound weight loss over the past couple of months. While denying a decreased need for sleep or insomnia, the family had also noted that she had been spending money excessively and exchanging sex for money. Amy reported smoking two to three cigarettes daily, using marijuana daily, and drinking one to two days per week. She denied recent cocaine or stimulant use, and her urine toxicology was positive only for THC.

On exam, Amy was noted to be bizarrely dressed, wearing an unkempt blonde wig, dark sunglasses throughout the interview, "dramatic" eye makeup, excessive lipstick, and tight-fitting female clothing. She had a tangential thought process, with noted persecutory and grandiose delusions, and preoccupations about the secret society. Her mood was "scared," her affect was labile, and her insight and judgment were impaired. Her medical workup included routine psychiatric labs and a head CT, which were all within normal limits. Amy was admitted to the inpatient psychiatric unit and initially treated with risperidone, which was titrated up to 4 mg at bedtime with an improvement in paranoid ideation and psychotic symptoms. Amy was discharged home with a diagnosis of schizophreniform disorder given the short duration of symptoms.

Amy was sent to the emergency room again a week later by her outpatient psychiatrist due to recurrent psychotic symptoms, mood lability, ideas of reference, and vocalizing a need to leave the family in order to join the secret society. When questioned about her plan to join the secret society, she stated that her plan was to begin walking aimlessly until she was "found" by them. Amy was again admitted to the inpatient psychiatric unit, and due to the ongoing mood lability and concern for bipolar illness, Amy was started on lithium and titrated up to 1200 mg. She remained in the hospital for 3 weeks, and risperidone was cross-taped to olanzapine, with significant improvement in both mood and psychotic symptoms. Amy was diagnosed with schizoaffective disorder and discharged home to family. She was seen in the emergency room once more the following week for ongoing delusions and plans to leave and join the secret society; however, she was evaluated and discharged back home.

Over the next couple of years, Amy was seen in outpatient treatment and treated with aripiprazole and escitalopram for her diagnosis of schizoaffective disorder and GD. She was seen in a combination of individual therapy in a dynamic, open-ended frame and medication management on a weekly basis. She continued to express her desire for estrogen, and given her history of GD, and the relative stability of her psychiatric symptoms, she was started on estrogen with careful monitoring from her entire treatment team. In many ways, she understood that her psychiatric treatment was a requirement for ongoing hormonal care and was motivated to attend her sessions to ensure she was able to access care.

Through her treatment, Amy maintained a strong and consistent gender identity. Amy maintained an intense desire and insistence to be a woman and consistently attended sessions with long hair, makeup, and female attire. She spoke frequently about her desire to have gender reassignment surgery and wanting to "have it off" in reference to her male genitalia. She was noticeably distressed during a session in which she did not have time to shave her face prior to arriving and endorsed high levels of discomfort and embarrassment about having male secondary sex characteristics. She also frequently made reference to her role as an older sister to her sibling and her role in the strong female lineage in the family. She spoke frequently about opening a "new chapter" following her gender reassignment surgery and talked with enthusiasm her ability to wear lower-cut shirts and skirts if she desired.

In the middle of the year with her current treatment provider, Amy began to report increasing depression, fatigue and hypersomnia, irritability, and anxiety. During this time, she was also noted to be consistently more distressed and tearful in session, along with an increase in the volume and veracity of delusional content. Her clinical picture at this time was complicated by concurrent marijuana use and suspected alprazolam abuse by the family. Due to concern for an episode of bipolar depression, along with ongoing side effects of sedation from aripiprazole, aripiprazole was cross-tapered to lurasidone with significant improvements in mood, sedation, and a decrease in delusional content to baseline levels.

Throughout the year, content of individual sessions frequently centered around feelings of being "stuck" in life, especially in terms of employment and romantic relationships. It was noted that since treatment at the beginning of the year, there had been little conversation about her gender reassignment surgery, which had been the initial stated goal at the beginning of the year. Following a discussion with both Amy and her family, a surgical consult was scheduled with improvements in her mood and future orientation.

During the latter part of the year, Amy endured a sexual assault resulting in a significant suicide attempt by overdose on her prescribed hormones and psychiatric medications. Following evaluation in the emergency room, she was admitted for a brief inpatient hospitalization and restarted on her medications.

Throughout treatment, Amy would frequently reminisce about her life as a gay male, commenting on how much she enjoyed her party lifestyle and popularity during those years. It was reflected back to Amy that this was also a time of greater acceptance of her gender identity, from her friends, her family, her romantic relationships, and to society in general. Amy's ongoing delusions were conceptualized as fantasy to escape the struggles of not only an individual with a mental illness but also being a transgender individual. By scheduling her surgical consult, Amy felt a needed sense of acceptance from her family of her gender identity as a female. Although she continued to endorse delusions throughout her treatment that varied in severity based upon mood symptoms and concurrent substance use, her stated gender identity remained constant throughout her treatment course. At this point, she is scheduled for her gender-affirming surgery under close watch from her family and her outpatient treatment team.

Notably, family members were involved throughout her treatment, with the primary family intervention being psychoeducation about GD and transgender issues along with the chronicity and stability of psychotic delusions. Amy's family was also very proactive in exploring community volunteer opportunities, supportive employment, and support groups through NAMI.

Case Discussion

Many studies have shown that transgender individuals face significant amounts of discrimination, harassment, violence, and family rejection. Members of the LGBT community, and especially transgender individuals, face a high degree of what is termed "minority stress." These factors play a tremendous role in the development and maintenance of psychopathology. Independent of this, GD is present across all societies, ethnicities, and backgrounds, and individuals with GD are not spared affliction with co-occurring psychiatric illnesses, including chronic psychotic illnesses such as schizophrenia and schizoaffective disorder. Unfortunately, the literature is limited on best approaches for individuals with both GD and psychotic illness, and, as a result, these individuals are often denied access to care.

For Amy, since her initial evaluation in the specialized gender service, she had come to understand herself as a woman and met full diagnostic criteria for GD. Diagnostically, prior to referring for either hormones or surgery, it was important to track Amy's symptoms of GD during her multiple emotional states. Due to the chronic nature of her psychotic illness, and her frequent experience of relapse of symptoms, there were multiple opportunities to assess her experience of her gender both during times of stability and times of overt psychosis. It is the consistent presence of GD across illness states that ultimately allowed her treatment providers to feel confident in connecting her to medical and surgical care for her GD. For Amy, when she was able to articulate clear understanding and insight into her psychotic symptoms, she experienced GD. When she was in the throes of psychosis and believed to the core of her being that she could wander the streets and be picked up by a secret society, she experienced GD. In many ways, her GD became the most consistent part of her experience, and regardless of illness state, she had a clear and consistent desire to medically and surgically transition and even in her most psychotic states could still clearly articulate the risks and benefits of the choices in her care.

As such, the challenge for the outpatient treatment providers was not if hormones or surgery would be appropriate but how to manage it safely. As it turns out, the hormones made no significant impact on her psychotic symptoms, but it did make her feel more whole and more comfortable in her body and her identity. Surprisingly, one of the biggest challenges was about the structural barriers to accessing care. As a part of her relapsing illness, Amy would often disappear from treatment and have difficulties in remembering follow-up visits. Some clinicians might interpret these missed appointments as possible unconscious ambivalence to treatment, and that was discussed as a possibility; however, it was clear with ongoing treatment that it was better explained as a primary failure in executive functioning due to her psychotic illness. Thus, the treatment team had to take a primary role in helping Amy to structure her weeks and put into place home-based resources to help her access the care she so desired and needed.

Conclusion

Amy has a chronic and severe mental illness that will persist throughout her life. She also happens to be a transgender woman with a tremendous number of strengths and a confidence in her sense of self and wishes for her future. Historically, her psychotic symptoms would have barred her from accessing gender-affirming care, and certainly they complicated her treatment course but often in ways that were unexpected. There was an appropriate balance of caution and advocacy for her care throughout, even though at times it was unclear if things were moving too quick or too slow. However, we found that if we used the basic ethical principles of autonomy, beneficence, non-malfeasance, and justice as a frame for treatment, it became much more straightforward on how to proceed.

Regarding autonomy, does an individual, even an individual who has a hard time differentiating reality from fantasy, have specific understanding about the risks, benefits, and alternatives of a medical intervention? Do they have capacity to consent to the specific interventions at hand? Is there wish for care consistent across disease states? If the answer is yes, regardless of psychotic symptoms, then they have a right to autonomy. Does gender-affirming care help the patient, fulfilling the ethical principle of beneficence? We know that accessing gender-affirming care improves quality of life and diminishes GD, and without evidence to the contrary, we can assume that it will also benefit those with psychotic symptoms. As for non-malfeasance, or the concept of doing no harm, we must build a more robust evidence base—there is no compelling evidence that estrogen or testosterone at usual treatment doses is any more dangerous to those with severe mental illness; however, there is also no compelling evidence that it is safe. There is simply no evidence either way. Which finally brings us to justice—the right to equal access of care. It is this ethical principle that has been most disregarded for individuals with severe psychotic illness. To be just in our care means to advocate for our patients who are unable to advocate for themselves and to get them access to care that is beneficial and necessary, even if it is at times controversial.

References

1. Murad MH, Elmain MB, Garcia MZ, Mullan RJ, Murad A, Erwin PJ, et al. Hormonal therapy and sex reassignment: a systematic review and meta-analysis of quality of life and psychosocial outcomes. Clin Endocrinol (Oxf). 2010;72:214–31.
2. Randell JB. Transvestitism and transsexualism: a study of 50 cases. Br J Psychiatry. 1959;2:1448–52.
3. Lukianowicz N. Transvestite episodes in acute schizophrenia. Psychiatry Q. 1962;36:44–54.
4. Dhejne C, Van Vlerken R, Heylens G, Arcelus J. Mental health and gender dysphoria: a review of the literature. Int Rev Psychiatry. 2016;28(1):44–57.
5. Bower H. The gender identity disorder in the DSM-IV classification: a critical evaluation. Aust N Z J Psychiatry. 2001;35:1–8.
6. Pope H, Katz D. Affective and psychotic symptoms associated with anabolic steroid use. Am J Psychiatr. 1988;145:487–90.
7. Costa R, Colizzi M. The effect of cross-sex hormonal treatment on gender dysphoria individuals' mental health: a systematic review. Neuropsychiatr Dis Treat. 2016;12:1953–66.
8. Grigoriadis S, Seeman MV. The role of estrogen in schizophrenia: implications for schizophrenia practice guidelines for women. Can J Psychiatr. 2002;47(5):437–42.
9. Meijer J, Eeckhout GM, van Vlerken RH, de Vries AL. Gender dysphoria and co-existing psychosis: review and four case examples of successful gender affirmative treatment. LGBT Health. 2017;4:2.

Chapter 13
Gender Dysphoria and Multiple Co-occurring Psychiatric Issues: Compare and Contrast

Rebecca A. Hopkinson and Nathaniel G. Sharon

Introduction

This chapter will focus on two cases of adolescents with gender dysphoria and co-occurring mental health conditions. Cody's case will illustrate (1) an adolescent with significant mental health conditions that were stable enough to progress with physical interventions for gender dysphoria and (2) treatment of his gender dysphoria and gender-related social supports improved his co-occurring mental health conditions. Sam's case will illustrate (1) an adolescent with co-occurring mental health conditions that could not be stabilized enough to safely begin medical treatments for gender dysphoria and (2) required treatment planning that focused on reducing the severity of his co-occurring mental health conditions prior to treatment for gender dysphoria.

These cases highlight the following clinical questions:

1. Why is screening for gender dysphoria and the social stressors related to gender diversity critical for assessment, diagnosis, and treatment planning?
2. Why is it clinically helpful to distinguish between symptoms arising from environmental stressors related to being gender diverse versus symptoms related to co-occurring conditions?
3. How should gender dysphoria be prioritized in treatment planning when there are co-occurring mental health conditions that are not well controlled?
4. Under what circumstances would interventions for gender dysphoria be put on hold in order to improve co-occurring conditions first?

R. A. Hopkinson, MD (✉)
Department of Psychiatry and Behavioral Sciences, Seattle Children's Hospital, University of Washington, Seattle, WA, USA
e-mail: rah2117@gmail.com

N. G. Sharon, MD
Division of Child and Adolescent Psychiatry, Department of Psychiatry and Behavioral Sciences, University of New Mexico, Albuquerque, NM, USA
e-mail: nsharon@salud.unm.edu

A. Janssen, S. Leibowitz (eds.), *Affirmative Mental Health Care for Transgender and Gender Diverse Youth*, https://doi.org/10.1007/978-3-319-78307-9_13

Brief Literature Review

Prior to an adolescent starting medical interventions for gender dysphoria, medical providers work hand-in-hand with mental health providers to assess the youth's gender development and needs as well as their emotional, psychological, social, and cognitive well-being to assure the best outcome for the youth [1]. The World Professional Association for Transgender Health Standards of Care [2] recommends medical, psychological, and the social problems are "well controlled" to start interventions and not interfere with treatment. The phrase "well controlled" can be difficult to interpret for mental health providers as there is a large degree of subjectivity. Some youth may present with no active concerns apart from gender dysphoria and have immensely supportive systems within their home and school environments. On the opposite end of the spectrum, other youth may present with severe substance use and mental health problems independent of gender dysphoria that severely interfere with the youth's ability to participate in the informed consent process and care plan. Youth may also have poor social support systems, whereby pursuing hormone therapy could potentially worsen their exposure to social risks such as physical violence at school or family rejection and even homelessness. For youth in emotional distress related to lack of family acceptance or school bullying, a clinician may need to offer psychoeducation and family therapy to the family and/or advocate within the school setting to help alleviate adjustment symptoms. If gender dysphoria is present, delaying or lack of treatment with hormones can worsen a youth's emotional distress and lead to depression, anxiety, and self-harm, yet complex factors also need to be taken into account as embarking on a phenotypic gender transition can be a challenging developmental task, even for the most "stable and supported" adolescents. A thorough assessment is vital to parsing out what aspects of the presenting symptoms may be environmentally related, specific to gender dysphoria, and/or attributable to an independent mental health condition.

Youth presenting for gender-related services in medical settings have been shown to have high rates of depressive and anxiety disorders, autism spectrum disorder, post-traumatic stress disorder, eating disorders, suicidal ideation and attempts, self-harm, and reduced global functioning [3–5]. The higher rates of mental health problems have been associated with minority stress [6], which is a term used to describe the mental health impacts of structural discrimination and stigma. A few studies have followed youth throughout the course of treatment for gender dysphoria and have shown improved psychological well-being associated with gender-affirming treatments [7, 8], suggesting some aspects of their presenting psychopathology was related to the internal factors related to the incongruence that characterizes gender dysphoria.

With data suggesting mental health conditions may improve with treatment of gender dysphoria, it is vital to understand the complex factors involved in the adolescent's presentation. Some youth present with independent psychopathology adding complexity to the treatment planning given challenges that may exist in accurately diagnosing gender dysphoria in addition to navigating the potential complexity of gender transition in this already difficult stage of development. In clinical situations where only one other co-occurring mental health condition is present, although still complex, determining the direction of causality between the gender dysphoria and associated mental health diagnosis can be challenging. In some situations presence of a co-occurring condition can make diagnosing gender dysphoria and/or understanding whether or not an individual is capable of moving forward with irreversible treatments more challenging. Most obvious would be the cases of psychosis, mania, or other conditions impairing capacity for informed assent to treatments. Other psychiatric conditions may impair the youth's decision-making processes, cognitive/social functioning, and/or global functioning in some way. However, when the adolescent presents with *multiple psychiatric co-occurring* conditions, then it can complicate the clinical presentation to an even more challenging degree. Therefore, the clinician must understand when to prioritize treatment of these co-occurring mental health challenges in order to accurately and safely move forward with treatments for gender dysphoria, which often have irreversible effects on the body. This chapter presents two cases, both with multiple co-occurring psychiatric conditions and gender dysphoria, to illustrate how the psychiatrist or clinician can move forward addressing one issue at a time.

Case 1: Sam

Sam is a 15-year-old individual assigned female at birth, who was seen in the substance abuse clinic and by the dialectical behavioral therapy treatment team. It was in this context he expressed his male identity to his therapist and was referred for a gender-informed assessment.

Sam had presented for services to the psychiatric clinic on several different occasions over the years for a variety of reasons. These included evaluations for gender dysphoria, bipolar disorder, oppositional defiant disorder, substance abuse, recurrent suicidality and self-harm, severe anxiety and OCD symptoms, and ADHD. Sam also had social difficulties and cognitive rigidity; thus, autism spectrum disorder was also considered as a diagnosis. While the presenting concerns were varied, a large contributing factor was the level of conflict between the teen and parents, frequently resulting in crises and calls to the therapist or the police. The range of conflict and consequences included verbal altercations, accusations of abuse, being kicked out of multiple schools, running away from home, and severe emotional dysregulation, all of which made the assessment for gender dysphoria and how to best plan for a safe gender transition complex and difficult.

Psychiatric History

Sam's treatment history prior to age 15 was extensive. He was behaviorally dysregulated from a very early age and was diagnosed with ADHD at age 5. He was prescribed stimulants requiring very high doses, which initially led to improvement but then eventually led to significant irritability. Based on this pattern, his treating doctor had suggested at age 9 that he might have bipolar disorder and was started on an atypical antipsychotic. He was then evaluated by a psychiatrist with expertise in bipolar disorder, and it was concluded that Sam did not at that time meet criteria for bipolar disorder and thus was taken off the atypical. He was continued on rotating high-dose stimulants throughout childhood and into adolescence.

When Sam presented to the psychiatry clinic at age 15, it was primarily in the context of making suicidal statements, emotional dysregulation, and oppositional behavior. On evaluation, he was diagnosed with major depression and started on an SSRI, and his stimulant was changed from one stimulant preparation to another in an attempt to find a lower dose that would be therapeutic. Attempts to decrease stimulants were met with resistance from parents, who were desperate for improvement. Attempts to use different medications were met with refusal from Sam, because of multiple prior trials with poor response and negative side effects.

He remained impulsive and hyperactive, often appearing giddy and silly. Sam also endorsed severe anxiety and OCD symptoms. He reported significant anxiety particularly in the social realm. He also reported contamination fears—for example, an unwillingness to come into contact with the toilet for fear of contamination. He would not share food with others due to fear of contamination from saliva.

Sam had difficulty maintaining friendships. He was frequently rejected by peers due to his limited ability to appropriately read and respond to social situations and cues, as well as odd and frequently offensive behavior. There was concern for autism spectrum disorder, although he had been evaluated as a child and it was ruled out at that time.

By age 15, Sam was using marijuana and alcohol. Sam's substance use terrified his parents, as Sam's aunt, who had also been diagnosed with bipolar disorder, had died of suicide after years of substance abuse. Sam was pre-contemplative regarding cessation throughout his treatment in the psychiatry clinic. His substance use progressively escalated and affected his functioning and safety as his behavior became more erratic, including staying out all night in the downtown of a metropolitan area, bringing substances to school, and not returning home or taking his medication.

Gender Development History

Since the age of 3 years old, Sam never presented as a typical female. His parents reported that he did not want to wear girl clothes or colors or do stereotypical "girl things." He played with both male and female peers, but struggled socially throughout life, rarely being able to keep friends of either gender. Sam enjoyed playing sports as a child, but preferred co-ed teams, as he reported that this helped him to feel that he was not perceived as female by others. It is unclear whether or not the other children did in fact perceive him to be male, but in his mind he felt he could blend in. When he was enrolled by his parents into an all-girls team, he refused to join, as he felt this would "out" him as female. He did attempt once as a child to present fully as male in one context, but once the other children discovered his assigned sex, they bullied him.

Sam had been evaluated at age 10 for gender dysphoria, but at that time he did not clearly articulate a need to change his body, and thus clinicians recommended "watchful waiting" (giving him time to see how his identity would evolve as he got older without transitioning to another gender), which was also preferred by his parents. This decision was influenced by his developmental age and his inability to consider medical treatment or his future at that time. In middle school, with the onset of puberty, he started to demonstrate more stereotypical feminine behaviors. For example, he tried out more feminine clothing and dated boys (which according to him was more of a "girl thing" to do) and even wore a dress in a school play. His parents felt that they had "dodged a bullet." However, in high school, Sam's gender identity concerns returned. Sam expressed his feelings of being male directly to his therapist at age 15 when he learned about puberty blockers from the Internet on Tumblr.

Psychosocial Factors

Sam's family often communicates in a highly reactive way, and there is a high level of conflict. His parents also struggled with impulsivity and emotional dysregulation. His father reported regretfully that he had difficulty managing his anger and had hit Sam as a child. His mother worked a high-level job with a lot of travel requirements and thus had limited time and engagement at home. His parents struggled to set appropriate limits, often reacting harshly, and then would not follow through with consequences. As a teenager, Sam and his family would have frequent physical altercations where his parents would report that he was out of control, hitting or threatening other family members, and on a few occasions subsequently required physical restraint by his father. During violent verbal and physical altercations, either Sam or his parents would frequently call the police, and Sam would report allegations toward his family. This led to the involvement of child protective services on a number of occasions; however, the allegations were determined to be unfounded.

On the other hand, Sam demonstrated some strengths. Sam is highly intelligent, musically gifted, and motivated by participation in the arts. Despite these strengths, he struggled to remain in school and was expelled from one alternative school after another. The reasons were multiple, including substance use in school, vandalizing school property, and sexual harassment of other students. He would make sexually provocative comments and drawings and once sent a sexually provocative letter to a female peer. His parents were supportive of finding the best fit for him, but even in a highly supportive, LGBT-friendly school environment, he failed to follow basic expectations.

Mental Status Exam

Sam was of slight stature and had short, straight black hair partially shaved on the sides of his head. His gender presentation was androgynous. He dressed in loose-fitting, ripped jeans, and a t-shirt from an obscure band. He made intermittent eye contact, sometimes furtive or avoidant, depending on the topic and the anxiety he experienced. He would easily grow oppositional and argumentative with parents, although cooperated well with the physician. He jiggled his leg constantly. His speech was rapid and at times the pitch and tone would increase when he was angry or highly emotional. His thought process was concrete, rigid, and with black and white thinking. When angry or anxious, his speech would increase in speed and volume. When in the midst of a conflict, his thinking became rigid, obsessive, and perseverative. He would often deny suicidal ideation, and stated when he makes suicidal statements to his parents, it is with the goal of getting them to attend to his needs and wants or to get back at them/upset them. He demonstrated no evidence of psychosis and no homicidal ideations or intent. If asked to state his mood, his response would simply be, "I'm just not happy." His affect appeared depressed, angry, and anxious and was congruent with mood. His impulse control was poor and was frequently observed to speak without forethought while laughing inappropriately. His insight was often rather poor. While he was aware of his own mood variations, severe anxiety, social difficulties and difficulties encountered with trialing multiple medications, he still struggled with his ability to see his role in conflict and have insight into other's perspectives. His judgment was poor. While being able to advocate for his own treatment, he struggled greatly with judging safety and surroundings.

DSM Diagnoses

From his prior history and initial assessment, Sam was given initial diagnoses of gender dysphoria, major depressive disorder, generalized anxiety disorder, obsessive-compulsive disorder, cannabis use disorder, alcohol use disorder, and parent-child relational problem. We considered probable diagnoses of social anxiety disorder, bipolar disorder, ADHD, unspecified trauma disorder, and autistic spectrum disorder as well.

Biopsychosocial Formulation

Sam initially presented with a long-standing history of ADHD and gender dysphoria, but also with a variety of symptoms including depression, anxiety, obsessions and compulsions, poor social skills, oppositional behavior, marijuana and alcohol use, and extreme familial conflict. Many diagnoses were considered, and many remained in question despite multiple years of treatment and assessment. For example, a long-standing diagnosis of ADHD that he appeared to meet criteria for as a child, and stimulants seemed to help at times, was not very clear at the time he presented in adolescence. After thorough history taking, it became clear that medication treatment of ADHD did not alleviate this child's suffering and deficits, and may have exacerbated his mood disorder, making it difficult to tease out whether they were co-occurring conditions or a misdiagnosis. Given the gender identity concerns, perhaps the additional element of a possible incongruence that characterizes gender dysphoria made the "ADHD vs. mood disorder vs. both" diagnostic considerations that much more difficult. However, Sam displayed chronic mood dysregulation and anxiety that appeared independent of gender dysphoria. Emotional dysregulation and anxiety symptoms occurred in many different environments and contexts, not just around gender identity/expression or social-related gender concerns. He had a significant family history for bipolar disorder, substance use, and suicide, making him more at risk for development of primary mood and substance use disorders. He also had a history of early childhood trauma, making him more prone to problems with emotional control and attachment. Psychologically, he was noted to do better when supported with appropriate limit setting and consistent, calm, validating responses by adults. His parents struggled with these skill sets and would often exacerbate symptoms through inconsistent and invalidating responses. He also had chronic low self-worth due to his difficulty with self-regulation, and he struggled to see how his behaviors impacted others. Sam displayed cognitive rigidity, resulting in arguing and conflict with family and occasionally treatment providers, peers, and teachers. Socially, Sam struggled with forming age-appropriate healthy social relationships and had difficulty eliciting positive responses from others, due to his inability to understand social interactions, which was not helped by the challenging environment in which he grew up. He spent most of his upbringing with his father, with whom he had the most conflict, due to mother working and not being present. The constant family conflict resulted in multiple crises, making healthy relationship-building skills in his life of any kind extremely difficult. Due to his limited emotional and social skills, he was expelled from multiple schools, resulting in limited positive social interactions and no friends. He experienced some bullying related to his gender diverse presentation, but over time it became clear that this was not the main cause of his social challenges. One potential factor contributing to his externalizing behaviors was that they may have been an attempt to demonstrate hyper-masculinity, perhaps due to his own insecurities and inadequacies with an unconscious understanding of how his lack of male anatomical features played a role in his ability to feel whole.

Treatment Course

Sam was admitted to the DBT program within the psychiatry clinic based on his complex presentation, his challenges with emotion regulation, conflict within the family, and his suicidal statements. During DBT treatment, Sam disclosed his male gender identity to his therapist as a primary stressor in his life. He chose to disclose this when he learned through the Internet that one could take hormone blockers in order to prevent puberty. He urgently wanted to pursue this option and was disappointed to learn that he had already progressed through puberty. He expressed a feeling of helplessness and hopelessness with regard to pursuing a gender transition, as he did not believe that his parents would support him, based on their failure to use preferred pronouns consistently and their relief when he briefly attempted to express himself in a more feminine way in middle school.

His parents were wary of a gender transition, feeling that the burden of the decision was on them, as they did not see their child as having the maturity and flexibility to weigh all the risks and benefits. Consistent with this belief, in many areas of his life, Sam did in fact display cognitive rigidity and black and white thinking. His poor judgments and impulsive behaviors were highly concerning to his parents, particularly with respect to his making such an important and complex decision to change his body irreversibly.

Sam was evaluated for gender dysphoria, and it was concluded that he did meet the criteria. It was also clear that he had presented a consistent, long-standing wish to be of the other gender and was requesting medical intervention. Sam had made a social gender transition at school, where peers used his preferred male pronouns and name. His parents were encouraged to also use his preferred name and pronouns, and efforts were made to help them grieve and accept Sam's gender as male, considering it had been long-standing and had not wavered. The goal of medical intervention was discussed with parents and the treatment team, with a plan to refer for hormone therapy. This referral was contingent on Sam's ability to comply with the necessary steps to participate in a medical intervention. He was asked to demonstrate continued, consistent participation in/presenting for psychotherapy, medical appointments, DBT group, and compliance with medications as prescribed. The expectation to maintain a basic level of psychiatric functioning was also recommended which included no psychiatric hospitalizations, abstention from self-injurious behaviors, impulsive suicidal behaviors in response to more trivial triggers, expulsions from school, the need for police calls to the home, and steps toward the treatment of substance use.

Concurrently, Sam and his parents were enrolled in the DBT program, where providers were affirming of transgender youth. They were coached on interpersonal effectiveness, emotion regulation skills, and mindfulness. Sam's parents made slow progress toward providing a more peaceful environment. In this context, they were encouraged to accept Sam's gender as part of providing a validating environment.

Despite making these steps toward the gender transition that was Sam's goal, Sam's psychiatric functioning continued to decline. It was difficult for Sam to experience the progress his parents were making due to the long history of conflict and lack of trust within the family. It is possible that his having to wait for his desired hormone therapy exacerbated his presentation; however, other factors also appeared to worsen independently. He frequently skipped school. He came to school with marijuana, which resulted in suspension. He continued to have conflict with his parents, and chose to run away from home repeatedly, staying out all night in the city or staying at homeless youth shelters. He would obtain money and shelter from other families by accusing his parents of abuse in order to gain sympathy. His behaviors were very concerning to his parents and treatment team as he appeared to have no insight into the dangerousness of his behavior.

He was intermittently adherent to medication due to his frequent periods of running away and lack of ability for his parents to provide adequate oversight. He missed psychotherapy sessions and DBT group, although he did consistently show up for his psychiatry appointments. He continued to voice suicidality to parents when they attempted to set limits.

One sizeable barrier to treating Sam's mental illness, and thus allowing for appropriate treatment of gender dysphoria, was the family's relationship to medications. Parents were highly resistant to remove or lower medications, particularly stimulants, due to being desperate for something to help Sam. While Sam was willing to trial removal of medications, he was appropriately reticent to try anything new, as he had felt like a test subject in his childhood due to constant medication changes and an aggressive regimen to "fix" him and his behavior. Thus, he remained on a combination of high-dose stimulants and an SSRI despite continuing to have frequent crises and limited to no benefit from the medications.

He was noted by teachers at times to appear elevated, talking fast, thinking fast, and giddy, as well as impulsive and inappropriate. One teacher described that he appeared to be high on stimulant medication, but his urine toxicology at the time only showed his prescribed methylphenidate. Based on this behavior, he was admitted to the psychiatric hospital with the intention to do a medication washout, as effect of the stimulants and SSRIs were of concern. He was transferred to a residential facility to provide further evaluation and stabilization, during which time he was diagnosed with bipolar disorder based on his continued elevated mood, and started on lithium.

However, when he returned home, his acting out behavior continued. He ran away from home and dropped out of treatment. It was determined that he was staying at friends' houses, thus obtaining food, shelter, and money. During this time he was using marijuana daily and heavily. Parents were able to locate him by reaching out to other parents and managed to pick him up and impose an admission to a long-term rehab. According to his parents, he is now much more emotionally stable and remorseful of his substance-related behavior, and grateful to his parents for continuing to pursue treatment for him, despite his resistance.

Case 2: Cody

Cody is a 17-year-old male (assigned female sex at birth) who initially presented for care at an academic psychiatric hospital at age 14 due to suicidal ideation in the context of a severe episode of depression. He had multiple plans for suicide including a desire to hang himself and had been contemplating suicide for several months. His grades were dropping, and he was eating one meal per day at the time of presentation. His primary stressors included ongoing bullying at school related to his male gender presentation, severe distress over female physical sex characteristics perceived incongruent to his experienced gender, and fear about coming out as male to his dad. He had been initiated on leuprolide injections for gender dysphoria 4 months prior to psychiatric hospitalization by a pediatric endocrinologist in order to reduce severe distress over continued female pubertal changes and monthly menstrual cycles. During hospitalization, he was initiated on sertraline to treat depression, anxiety, and obsessive-compulsive disorder (OCD) symptoms and referred for follow-up with an outpatient psychiatrist who had experience working with gender diverse youth.

Psychiatric History

Cody had a history of moderate combined-type attention deficit hyperactivity disorder (ADHD), obsessive-compulsive disorder (OCD) , and deficits in receptive and expressive communication, dating back to around 7 years old. He had been in individual psychotherapy since age 7 for symptoms of ADHD and obsessive-compulsive behaviors (need for symmetry, need for color coordination, and cleaning compulsions). He had symptoms of depression that also started around this time that Cody retrospectively endorsed as related to gender identity concerns. Around age 13, he began to develop some mild externalized and oppositional behaviors at school related to bullying about his male gender presentation. He had no prior history of medication trials, psychiatric hospitalizations, or suicide attempts. He had no history of any alcohol or substance use disorders.

Gender Development History

Cody's mom had no exposures during pregnancy and was healthy throughout. He had a normal birth without complications. He was assigned female at birth and was raised socially as female. Per the patient's mother, Cody had always preferred male-typical clothing, play behaviors, and peers since early childhood. At age 7, Cody began to display oppositional behaviors and tantrums when required to wear female clothing, particularly dresses. He would frequently refuse to leave the house or attend an event if made to wear a dress. Due to communication deficits, Cody struggled to communicate his needs and would resort to displays of anger to communicate distress regarding presenting as female gender. Cody reported retrospectively that he began to think about his gender around age 8 or 9. He describes thinking he felt as though he had been assigned the wrong gender of female and wanted to be a boy. Female pubertal development began at age 11 or 12, and Cody described going through these changes as traumatic. He began to experience more psychological distress related to the incongruence between his experienced gender of male and his female sex traits. Cody began to want others to perceive him as he saw himself (male) and said the development of female puberty made this extremely difficult. He also endorsed female sex characteristics as not aligning with his own perception of being male. He recalls that his distress from these body changes became severe at age 13 with onset of menarche. He developed severe suicidal ideation and self-injurious behaviors due to distress over these unwanted physical changes. After discussion with his therapist, he came out to his mother about his male gender identity. His mother was supportive and helped him come out as male to family and peers when he started the 9th grade. He was started on puberty suppression (a GnRH analogue, leuprolide) to halt female pubertal changes by a pediatric endocrinologist. He found great relief from this intervention by cessation of menses and pubertal development, although felt the leuprolide worsened his depressive symptoms.

He began to request being called by the male name Cody and wanted others to use male pronouns. He also began to dress daily in male-typical clothing and wore a compression binder to flatten his chest tissue to be perceived as male by others. He would frequently get verbally and physically harassed and threatened by his peers, which he reports was due to his gender presentation since he had been previously known as female. In response, Cody would engage in escalated verbal altercations back with the peers, which resulted in Cody receiving more consequences by the school than the initial perpetrators of the bullying. Cody also attempted to use the male bathroom at school but due to the peer harassment in the bathroom, started to avoid use of the school bathroom all day. This resulted in Cody holding his urine and led to the development of recurrent urinary tract infections. Due to these recurrent infections, Cody developed compulsive genital washing behaviors out of concern he would be identified as female.

Psychosocial and Legal Factors

Cody was raised by his biological mother and father until their divorce when he was a young child. His mother retained legal primary custody, while his father had visitation rights every other weekend. His father moved to a different city in the state and Cody continued to visit. His mother re-partnered to Cody's stepfather, who was also supportive and affirming of Cody's male gender identity. Cody has both an older sister who is lesbian-identified and highly supportive of him and a younger half sister who is equally supportive. His older sister helped him with his coming-out process and would drive him to youth-based transgender support groups in the city. All of the family members supported Cody by using the name and pronouns of his gender. However, Cody had not yet come out to his biological father regarding his gender identity. While his father was always more supportive of Cody's more male-typical behavior and they frequently bonded over camping and sports, he had heard his father make homophobic remarks and was convinced his father would not accept him as male.

His family was from a middle-class socioeconomic background, and when leuprolide was denied by insurance, his parents were able to pay for it out of pocket. They also were able to afford a therapist who had experience in gender dysphoria but did not accept insurance.

Cody received special education services in high school for having ADHD and communication deficits. Despite communication limitations, Cody was highly extroverted and socially driven, easily making friends at school. He was frequently the victim of bullying and occasionally harassment from teachers. He would occasionally lose control of his temper in response to these actions and often received punishment (detention, suspension) from the school administration for his impulsive, verbally explosive reactions. He would also request to skip school due to difficulty using the male bathroom and the bullying. The school, city, and state had no formal protection policies or bullying policies for gender diverse and transgender youth. Cody had to rely on the support of his academic counselor and Mom, who was employed at his school, to help intervene and mediate. This advocacy placed in her a difficult position as she was also an employee of the school. Cody enjoyed playing basketball and previously had been on the female basketball team in middle school. He initially wanted to play basketball but was not allowed to due to regulations he play on the team of the sex of his birth certificate. In Cody's state, he would have been required to have surgery prior to being allowed to change his birth certificate sex, something that was not possible for Cody at the time.

Mental Status Exam

Cody initially presented as a shorter-statured, average weight adolescent in casual male attire, binding his chest so individuals could not see the presence of his breasts when he was close. He had meticulous hygiene and grooming with matching shoes and color coordination. His eye contact was variable, and although he was typically well-engaged in appointments, he was also shy. His speech was non-spontaneous, although he would actively reply to questions with brief, linear responses. His speech spontaneity improved throughout the course of the interview or session, which was likely due to his feeling more comfortable with the provider. He had no endorsement of psychosis and suicidal or homicidal thoughts although did have anxious ruminations about his gender expression and acceptance. He also endorsed thoughts to self-harm when feeling stressed. His mood was typically reported as "better," and his affect was restricted to the anxious and subeuthymic range. He had some mild motor fidgeting and grew distractible toward the end of the interview, with a demonstration of distractibility from small stimuli. His insight and judgment were both fair when not under stress or being bullied.

DSM Diagnoses

Cody's presenting diagnoses on evaluation were gender dysphoria of adolescence/adulthood, major depressive episode (severe, without psychotic features), unspecified obsessive-compulsive disorder, unspecified communication disorder, and attention deficit hyperactivity disorder (combined, moderate).

Biopsychosocial Formulation

Cody initially presented after psychiatric hospitalization for suicidal ideation with intent and severe depressive symptoms as well as anxious adjustment symptoms and compulsive hygiene behaviors. He met criteria for gender dysphoria of adolescence regarding the incongruence between his affirmed/experienced male gender being at odds with female sex characteristics. He was also struggling with environmental stressors of bullying and harassment from peers and staff at school as well as fear of rejection from his father if he came out as transgender. He was being maintained on leuprolide, a medication that stops all hormone production and might have potentially been contributing to worsened vegetative symptoms of depression (loss of energy and appetite, loss of motivation), despite its benefits to buy time prior to initiation of cross-sex/gender hormone administration which have more irreversible effects. Regardless, with pubertal suppression, Cody continued to have ongoing distress regarding breast tissue that had already developed and the lack of male sex characteristics. His compulsive hygiene behaviors were worsened by the acute stressors of depression as well as ongoing recurrent urinary tract infections. He was unable to use the male restroom due to school policies and bullying, leading to him hold his urine for extended periods and subsequent infections. He had ADHD and elements of receptive and expressive communication problems, making it more challenging for him to use verbal skills and have some impulse control for issues around coming out and for interfacing with peer and school staff harassment. He would instead more readily rely on immature coping strategies that included both externalized expressions of frustration and internalized self-injurious behaviors. He had positive support from his lesbian-identified older sister, other siblings, and all caregivers and a mom who was willing to advocate for him in medical and academic settings. His family was more financially well-off than other peers from his state and could afford behavioral health care and medication that was not covered by insurance. Recognizing the degree to which addressing his gender dysphoria through irreversible interventions such as testosterone, which would help masculinize his body and thus potentially increase the degree to which he is perceived as male, was important given his age (most non-gender dysphoric—or cisgender—males have entered or were well progressed into puberty by this time). This would need to be weighed against helping him develop more positive coping strategies to reduce the impulsivity and navigate the complex aspects of gender transition within this family climate (father not even knowing about his male identity) and other psychiatric co-occurring conditions (ADHD, OCD, self-injury).

Treatment Course

Cody continued outpatient services with a child psychiatrist and individual therapist. Care was coordinated carefully with his pediatric endocrinologist. His main goals of care were to (1) continue to pursue physical interventions for gender dysphoria, (2) increase support in school regarding his social transition, and (3) improve his coping strategies for dealing with distress from gender dysphoria and environmental stressors. He continued with sertraline for anxiety and depression. In therapy, he worked emotional regulation when facing discrimination and bullying and problem-solving skills. He and his therapist worked on reduction of self-injurious behaviors when stressed and ways to have more self-agency when feeling powerless over negative feelings. He continued to endorse anhedonia and loss of energy on leuprolide and was eager to progress to testosterone.

Prior to testosterone initiation, Cody identified he needed to better master two goals including improved skills and interventions for bullying and his handling of those situations (anger episodes and self-harm behaviors) as well as coming out to his father. He knew his physical appearance would change on testosterone, and therefore he would not be able to hide these changes from his peers at school or his father, both having awareness that he was born with an assigned female gender. His mother had full legal custody and medical decision-making rights for Cody, but the family wanted to include his father in this process as Cody would be eventually seeing him while physically changing on testosterone. The concern was that had Cody began undergoing a phenotypic gender transition without others knowing, it could potentially introduce further conflict with those (such as his father) who had not known that this was the lifelong direction he was headed in. We therefore arranged a phone session with his father that included and provided psychoeducation about gender dysphoria and the subsequent helpful interventions. This led his father to express support for Cody and support the use of testosterone that Cody thought were best for himself to feel comfortable. Cody was greatly relieved by this therapeutic intervention and found that the exploration of how to best come out was helpful. Self-injurious behavior ceased as a result of this alone. He continued to display some intermittent anger episodes at school, particularly when teachers would not believe him about bullying or would automatically side with his aggressors. However, overall his emotional regulation and communication skills improved. After collaboration with his pediatric endocrinologist to ensure he was at maximum height and extensive review with Cody and his family on the impacts of testosterone therapy, Cody started testosterone injections at age 15. He continued with leuprolide therapy as well.

Meetings were arranged at the school with his academic counselor, individual therapist, and child psychiatrist to provide psychoeducation on best practices for supporting Cody at school and to review response policies to bullying. Attempts were made at increasing supports for his gender transition and bullying by integrated gender-affirming supports into his individual education plan. Mom obtained an outside school advocate to help liaison with the school regarding their lack of response to the bullying episodes. Accommodations were made so that he could use the nursing restroom, which he desired to use considering he was not yet comfortable using the male restroom, and this helped reduce the rate of urinary tract infections.

With these interventions, the vast majority of Cody's mental health symptoms improved. His depression remained in remission and his compulsive hygiene washing ceased. He continued to have mild OCD tendencies but not to the point of functional impairment. He did require ongoing treatment for ADHD, which did not improve with care for gender dysphoria. An attempt to taper sertraline was mildly successful at first, but after a significant physical assault that then led to post-traumatic stress symptoms, sertraline use resumed. He continued to function and develop well in all emotional, cognitive, sexual, and social domains.

Case Discussion

The above cases highlight the complexities and different care routes the patient, family, and providers must take when considering treatment for gender dysphoria in the context of multiple co-occurring psychiatric conditions. The presence of these conditions alone should not preclude treatment for gender dysphoria according to the World Professional Association of Transgender Health Standards of Care [2]. However, the task of the child and adolescent psychiatrist is to understand the complex biopsychosocial factors that contribute to the presentation of every adolescent and understand the relationship between any co-occurring conditions and whether or not this impacts the ability to make an accurate diagnosis of gender dysphoria and in addition determine the eligibility *and* readiness for such interventions.

For Sam, his emotional dysregulation and substance use impaired his life functioning to the point that treatments for gender dysphoria were placed on hold until he was more consistently sober and displaying improved mastery of his emotional and cognitive skills. Conversely, with Cody, it was determined that addressing the co-occurring psychiatric issues and enhanced social advocacy efforts could lead to quicker treatment for gender dysphoria, which led to a reduction of his presenting symptoms.

While Sam met criteria for gender dysphoria, and by the time he left care for residential substance abuse treatment, both Sam and his parents were of the mindset that he should receive treatment for his gender dysphoria. This change in parents' thinking took time to develop. Sam initially struggled with rigid, black and white thinking that impaired his ability for full understanding of hormone interventions and their longitudinal impact on his health and body. During acute treatment, Sam's mental health had deteriorated to the point that it was unlikely that he would have been able to follow through with the expectations and recommendations required for hormone therapy, nor would he be able to successfully manage the complexity of the social interactions that would take place as a result of his changing appearance in a healthy way. He would miss appointments and run away from home, making it impossible to provide consistent medical care. Sam struggled to coordinate with his parents, or even be in the same room with them, thus creating a barrier to obtaining treatments that require parental support, trust, participation, and consent. He also displayed severe mood vacillations that may have been exacerbated by substance use, frequently impairing both judgment and insight. Given the multiple barriers to care that impeded Sam's functioning, resulting in his being kicked out of multiple schools, running away, and constant conflict with family, Sam existed in a state of crisis, as did his family. These crises prevented Sam from being able to move forward in a consistent way in any area of his life, including working toward a gender transition.

While gender dysphoria may have been contributing to some of Sam's presenting symptoms, symptoms existed in multiple other contexts, and therefore it was concluded that his challenging presentation could not fully be attributed to gender dysphoria. Addressing gender dysphoria would have likely not addressed his primary mood and impulse control disorders that threatened his safety and well-being. His presentation was also due to a lack of functional skills on the part of both the parents and youth to emotionally regulate or navigate conflict in a functional manner. Likely, Sam would have continued to have poor functioning until obtaining treatment for his intense emotional dysregulation, poor impulse control, and substance use as well as being provided with family-based interventions.

Cody was able to more rapidly progress in treatment for gender dysphoria. Cody had multiple similar factors, including depression, OCD symptoms, and suicidality. A key difference in Cody's case was that many of his presenting symptoms were related to both his internal distress over sex/gender incongruence and environmental stressors related to his gender diversity (bullying). This was in direct contrast to Sam, whose presentation was not related to social sequelae of gender diversity or gender dysphoria. Sam lives in a liberal community where people are less likely to be bullied for a different gender expression than would be expected based on assigned sex at birth, and it does not appear that this is the reason that he was rejected by peers. Cody, as opposed to Sam, did not struggle with a severe substance use disorder or symptoms of bipolar disorder, both of which complicated Sam's case more intensely.

Initially, Cody's adaptive functioning was limited, and he would deal with stressors through anger outburst and self-harm. These limitations were worsened by his communication deficits and poorer executive functioning characterized by an ADHD diagnosis. He worked hard in individual therapy to improve these adaptive skills and better prepare himself for the social stressors he faced during his physical transition on hormones. Cody did require medication during the acute phase of treatment for depression and OCD symptoms and responded well to the medication. The gradual use of typical psychiatric interventions—both therapy and psychotropic medication—created a situation where better clarity regarding the timing of gender dysphoria treatment (testosterone) became apparent. The use of medication was helpful to support Cody to participate and learn effectively in therapy. Cody also stayed engaged in treatment because he was highly motivated to face the social challenges of gender transition and find ways to deal more effectively with each challenge. He continues to be at risk of intermittent periods of major depression and has continued ADHD symptoms into young adulthood. He remains active in his own behavioral health care and does not associate it with stigma or shame. While treatment gender dysphoria did not "cure" all his mental health conditions, it vastly improved his development in all areas and his overall psychological well-being. Helping Cody and his family appreciate that gender dysphoria (and its treatment) did not encompass his entire psychiatric presentation and future identity successfully allowed for Cody to move forward with addressing this important treatment intervention that would have hampered his psychological growth and development had it not been provided.

Sam and his family, on the other hand, struggled with following treatment recommendations, including attending appointments and taking or changing medications. Due to his lack of response to outpatient treatment, continued psychiatric decline, and increasingly dangerous behaviors, Sam's parents obtained more intensive treatment for Sam to address his mood and substance use. We remain hopeful that in the future, when his mental health problems are under control, Sam will be able to move forward with a plan that incorporates gender transition in a successful and healthy way, at a pace that addresses his many challenges, and does not bring more harm than good to his life.

When a youth with gender identity concerns presents with multiple co-occurring mental health concerns, considering the diagnosis of gender dysphoria and its treatments should not be left unaddressed or dismissed. Reviewing what the youth's goals are for the timing of their desired gender transition and supporting them toward these goals should always be part of the plan. However, the route and pace for proceeding forward can look different for each adolescent depending on what mental health issues present. Helping the youth and family decide together on prioritizing goals can be difficult to navigate depending on the complexity of the mental health problems and family dynamics. Fundamentally, if medical interventions are collaboratively deemed an effective way to alleviate the adolescent's distress, it is important for the youth to have the capacity to understand the basic indications, risks, benefits, and alternatives to the treatments and provide assent. In addition, the treatment goals should be tailored to promote the most optimal functioning and developmental outcomes for the youth. If stabilizing other mental health concerns, such as severe anorexia nervosa, substance use, acute self-injury, emotional dysregulation, etc., needs to first occur to optimize the functioning of the youth such that they can safely and successfully navigate the complexity of gender dysphoria treatment, this should guide the pace of the gender dysphoria treatment, all the while providing affirmation of the patient's wish to proceed more quickly. Ideally, both should be addressed at the same time if possible, as untreated gender dysphoria can lead to increase in depressive and anxious symptoms, so helping an adolescent understand that he/she is equally invested in addressing the gender-sex incongruence that characterizes gender dysphoria is crucial in developing trust and forming a therapeutic alliance.

How the provider conceptualizes the interaction between gender dysphoria and co-occurring psychopathology is extremely important, and absolute conceptualizations appear to be harmful. On one hand, attributing presenting psychopathology *exclusively* to a youth's gender identity concerns can emphasize that gender dysphoria treatment is the sole means of addressing the co-occurring psychopathology. On the other hand, conveying the message that a patient is psychiatrically compromised and thus ignoring their gender dysphoria can lead to a lack of appropriate validation and affirmation of gender dysphoria and lack of rapport which in turn may delay gender dysphoria treatment unnecessarily and affect one's ability to treat other presenting problems. While treatment of gender dysphoria and affirming gender practices can alleviate psychological distress, this does not mean that transgender youth cannot have primary mental health problems that cisgender youth also face. Attributing symptoms of bipolar disorder to distress from social stigma could place a youth at risk by not treating the underlying mood disorder. In Sam's case, regardless of gender dysphoria, he had other emotional regulation problems that needed urgent treatment.

Conversely, gender identity concerns should always be screened for and taken seriously when present, and gender dysphoria should be considered. Not addressing gender dysphoria can lead to "false negatives" in presenting patients, and then this could guide the treatment plan down an ineffective path. Both cases highlight the need for (1) screening for gender dysphoria for all youth; (2) understanding the importance of the pace and appropriateness of gender dysphoria management, regardless of the youths' goals of care; and (3) tailored approaches to treatment for gender dysphoria, depending on the severity of co-occurring mental health problems.

Conclusion

Supporting a youth, their family, and their medical providers when considering medical interventions for gender dysphoria should be a process tailored to each individual adolescent, particularly when multiple psychiatric co-occurring issues are at hand. Sam and Cody's cases illustrate how goals in care can vary depending on the severity of presenting mental health problems. Treatment plans should not be dictated by a set of prescribed pathways, but rather by the guidepost of supporting the youth toward their ultimate emotional, social, and cognitive development and functioning. Regardless of treatment plan, a youth should always be socially affirmed and acknowledged in their identified gender, as the lack of doing so can perpetuate symptoms of the co-occurring conditions and thus make the treatment course more difficult. This alone can help keep the youth engaged in care, reduce distress, and provide a safe space for mental health care.

References

1. Leibowitz S, Telingator C. Assessing gender identity concerns in children and adolescents: evaluation, treatments, and outcomes. Curr Psychiatry Rep. 2012;14:111–20.
2. Coleman E, Bockting W, Botzer M, Cohen-Kettenis P, DeCuypere G, Feldman J, et al. Standards of care for the health of transsexual, transgender, and gender-nonconforming people, version 7. Int J Transgenderism. 2011;13:165–232.
3. de Vries AL, Noens IL, Cohen-Kettenis PT, van Berckelaer-Onnes IA, Doreleijers TA. Autism spectrum disorders in gender dysphoric children and adolescents. J Autism Dev Disord. 2010; 40(8):930–6.
4. Costa R, Dunsford M, Skagerberg E, Holt V, Carmichael P, Colizzi M. Psychological support, puberty suppression, and psychosocial functioning in adolescents with gender dysphoria. J Sex Med. 2015;12(11):2206–14.
5. Connolly MD, Zervos MJ, Barone CJ 2nd, Johnson CC, Joseph CL. The mental health of transgender youth: advances in understanding. J Adolesc Health. 2016;59(5):489–95.
6. Carmel TC, Erickson-Schroth L. Mental health and the transgender population. J Psychosoc Nurs Ment Health Serv. 2016;54(12):44–8.
7. Spack NP, Edwards-Leeper L, Feldman HA, Leibowitz S, Mandel F, Diamond DA, et al. Children and adolescents with gender identity disorder referred to a pediatric medical center. Pediatrics. 2012;129(3):418–25.
8. de Vries ALC, McGuire JK, Steensma TD, Wagenaar ECF, Doreleijers AH, Cohen-Kettenis PT. Young adult psychological outcome after puberty suppression and gender reassignment. Pediatrics. 2014;134:2013–958.

Index

A. Janssen, S. Leibowitz (eds.), *Affirmative Mental Health Care for Transgender and Gender Diverse Youth*, https://doi.org/10.1007/978-3-319-78307-9

MIX
Papier aus verantwortungsvollen Quellen
Paper from responsible sources
FSC® C105338

If you have any concerns about our products,
you can contact us on
ProductSafety@springernature.com

In case Publisher is established outside the EU,
the EU authorized representative is:
Springer Nature Customer Service Center GmbH
Europaplatz 3, 69115 Heidelberg, Germany

Printed by Libri Plureos GmbH
in Hamburg, Germany